Stephen's Manual of EKG Interpretation:

A Concise Course

By Stephen M. Teich, M.D.

Dedicated to Susan, Elise, Brian and Andrew

With gratitude to my parents who provided the support and means for my education, to my instructors who filled my toolbox, to Dr. Martin N. Frank who enabled my clinical career, to all the colleagues, nurses and technicians with whom I have been privileged to work, and especially to my patients who placed their trust in me and challenged me with their questions.

Table of Contents

Chapter 1: Definition of the EKG..5

Chapter 2: The Anatomic and Physiologic Basics..............7

Chapter 3: The EKG Lead System..13

Chapter 4: Factors Influencing Wave Morphology............19

Chapter 5: The P Wave...28

Chapter 6: The QRS Complex..33

Chapter 7: Arrhythmias: Part 1 – Ectopic Type..................47

Chapter 8: Arrhythmias: Part 2 – Reentrant Type............63

Chapter 9: Heart Block..76

Chapter 10: Ischemic Patterns..82

Image credits...100

Index..101

About the author..103

Chapter 1: Definition of the Electrocardiogram (EKG)

The heart is a muscular organ that emits electromagnetic signals in three dimensions, the way a light bulb radiates lumens. It does so by the activation of embedded nerve tissue called the conduction system which normally follows a specific prescribed route. An electrocardiogram (EKG) is a tracing of these signals, recorded by placing cables on the body. From these, twelve leads are defined, each of which act as an individual observer of the heart from its unique angle. Twelve leads are useful to give one an appreciation of the three dimensional events on a two dimensional piece of paper.

The EKG provides us with the following information:

- It defines the heart's rhythm as normal or discloses abnormal variations called arrhythmias.

- It reflects the heart rate in beats per minute (bpm).

- It tells us of the health of the circuitry described above. Components may become diseased from age, drugs, infections or ischemia.

- The height and width of the signals can change with variations in the sizes and thickness of the four heart chambers from disease states.

-It can indicate if there is damage to the heart from previous infarctions and it can disclose if the heart is ischemic and in jeopardy of new damage.

- It gives clues if there are disturbances in body electrolytes, especially potassium.

Albert Einstein once said, "Everything should be made as simple as possible, but not simpler." The purpose of this book is to do just that with respect to the EKG. It starts by discussing basic anatomy and physiology, origin of the lead system and the way these interact with each other to create a tracing. After that, the specific events that occur with each heart beat will be explained in sequence, including pathologic conditions most frequently seen in the clinical practice of cardiology. The emphasis is on "Why?" as opposed to rote memorization. I try to anticipate the reader's questions as we proceed and address them in a way that keeps the narrative running smoothly.

Chapter 2: The Anatomic and Physiologic Basics

What follows is a series of discussions, each like a brick and self-contained, that together will be joined to give a foundation upon which an understanding of the EKG will be made easier in the subsequent chapters. Illustrations from the public domain (credit being cited with information, where available) and tracings from my personal collection will be utilized.

We start with basic anatomy and some physiology. If one never saw a picture of the heart before but heard a description, one would picture a simple square grid of four defining the two upper and two lower chambers: the right and left atria (RA and LA) above, and the right and left ventricles (RV and LV) below.

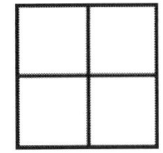

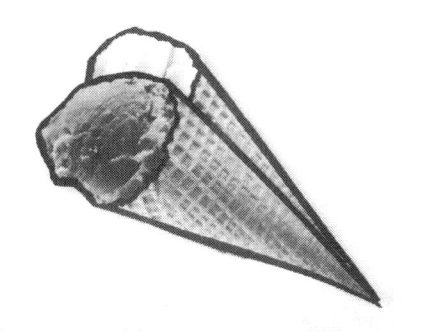

However, when facing a patient, the heart rests on the diaphragm with the atria positioned more to the right side of the ventricles than above them. The left side of the heart is predominantly posterior to the right, eclipsed with only its edge peeking out from the left lateral border. In the image below, Fig. 2, the chocolate ice cream is the RA, the vanilla the LA. The front cone is the RV covering much of the LV which is behind. In addition, the tips of the cones are pointed outward, off the plane of the page, tilting the atria toward the back, placing the LA furthest away from the chest surface, adjacent to the esophagus.

Another way to appreciate this is as follows: position your right hand in front of yourself, fingers widespread and pointing up. With palm facing left, place the thumb, up and down, flush against your sternum. Then pivot the hand about 30 degrees to the left. It is now in the plane of the heart's midline, defined by the ventricular and atrial septa, the walls that separate right chambers from left. Any structure in front of the hand is right heart; anything behind is left heart. The atria are on either side of the thumb, the ventricles on either side of the rest of the hand. They converge at the cardiac apex which is where the tip of your fifth finger's nail is: down, leftward and pointing forward. This explains why the PMI (point of maximal impulse) is felt just beneath the left breast on physical exam.

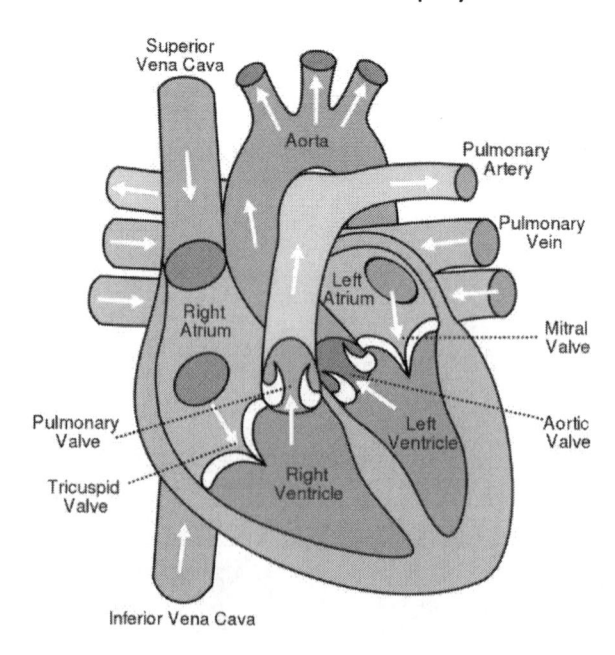

Fig. 3. Anatomy of the heart

Fig, 3 is a simple schematic of a heart. Notice the orientation and the fact that the anterior wall is removed to show the interior. In brief review, venous, deoxygenated blood returns from the body to the RA which allows it to drain to the RV below when the tricuspid valve is open. At the end of passive return the atrium contracts to boost the end filling volume of the right ventricle.

Next, the RV contracts and pumps blood to the lungs for oxygenation via the pulmonary arteries. This returns from the lungs via the pulmonary veins to the left atrium which, in similar fashion, allows the LV to fill by flow through the mitral valve, ending with left atrial contraction. The LV, now fully loaded, sends oxygenated blood to the body.

Of course, the process occurs simultaneously, in tandem, on both sides of the heart, the atria contracting together followed, after a short pause, by the ventricles. The filling phase of chambers is called diastole. The contraction of these muscular chambers is called systole and is made possible by the conduction system, a nerve network that conducts an electric current in a sequence designed to allow timing to be correct for a successful heart beat. Later, it will be seen that if an electrical block occurs in this path, the current can be conducted by the muscle tissue of the heart itself but not as quickly. The reason is that nerve tissue is covered by an insulator called myelin whereas myocardial tissue is not.

Fig. 4. Conduction system

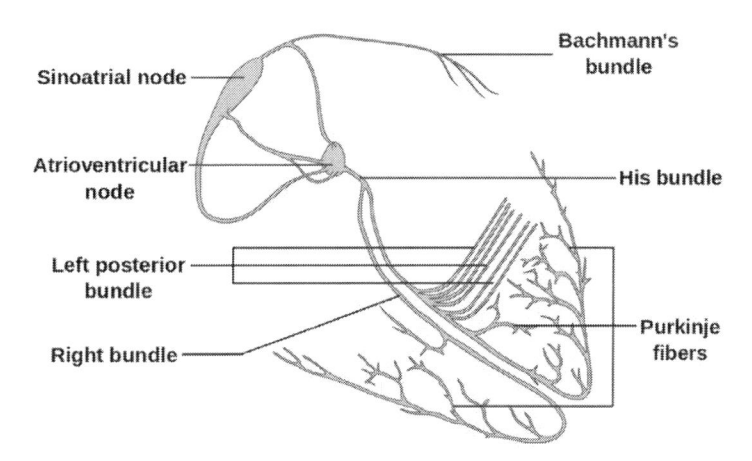

The above diagram, Fig. 4, shows the parallel orientation of the conduction system with the heart chambers because it is embedded within them.

The activation sequence is as follows:

The sinoatrial (SA) node is the normal pacemaker of the heart, normally sparking at 60 to 100 times a minute at rest in an adult. It is located in the right atrium (RA) at the upper right posterior corner where the superior vena cave joins that chamber. It fires repetitively because its cells are being collectively activated by action potentials which generate an electric charge due to the movement of charged ions across cell membranes.

The charge moves through nerve fibers of the RA which extend into the left atrium (LA) as well, through Bachmann's bundle, directed to the left and to the rear. This causes contraction of the two atria, sending blood to their respective ventricles below. Atrial contraction or systole is recorded as the P wave on the EKG. See fig. 5.

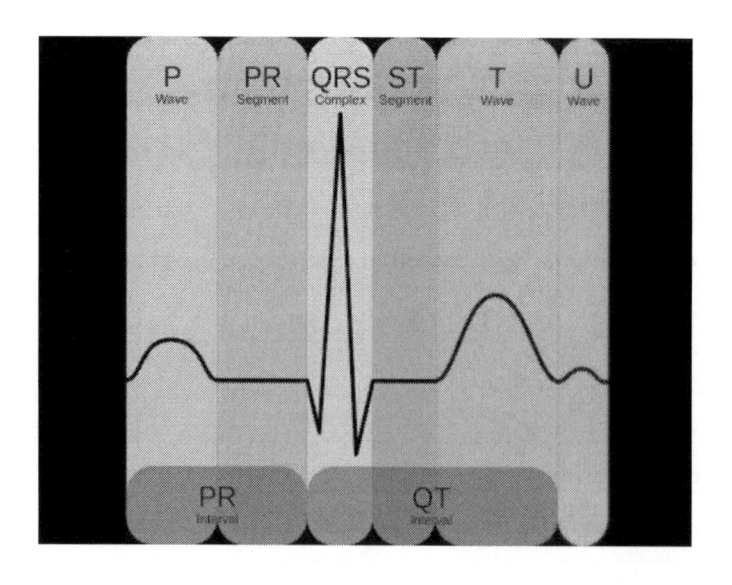

Fig.5. Waveform labels

The nerve fibers converge at the atrioventricular (AV) node which is located at a central point, near the intersection of all four cardiac chambers. The AV node conducts current but much more slowly than in the atria which gives time for the blood from atrial contraction to fill the ventricles before the latter are activated. The pause appears as a flat line on the EKG called the PR segment. The atria relax at this time but the relaxation signals are too small to affect the flat segment. The P wave plus the PR segment together are called the PR interval. It normally lasts between 120 and 200 milliseconds (msec). For future reference, anything named segment is flat; anything termed interval has vertical dimension and contains multiple components.

Leaving the AV node, the signal travels to the Bundle of His (also called the junction) which is a short trunk of nerve tissue that branches out, like a wishbone, into the right and left bundle branches (RBB and LBB). The Bundle of His can itself act as a pacemaker if the sinus node falters. Its intrinsic rate is 40 to 60 beats per minute (bpm) and such activity is called a junctional rhythm.

The bundle branches divide into the Purkinje fibers which bring the current to the two ventricles which contract, registering a QRS complex on the EKG. A QRS complex normally lasts about 80 msec. It is usually the tallest component of an EKG complex because it represents, for the most part, left ventricular activity. That chamber is the thickest of the four chambers with good reason. It must send blood from head to toe which requires a greater pressure than the right ventricle which only has to send blood locally to the lungs in the chest. For the same reasons the left bundle branch network feeding the LV is more extensive than the right bundle branch. The left has two branches (the anterior and posterior fascicles) as well as a branch that feeds the interventricular septum. Distal fibers can serve as yet another pacemaker if the sinus and junction fail, sitting in reserve, ready to fire at about 20 to 35 bpm, and termed idioventricular rhythm when it occurs.

Relaxation of the ventricles is physically passive and takes longer that active systole. It is represented by a flat ST segment and a mound called the T wave. A U wave is variably present and may represent relaxation of the left ventricle's papillary muscles which are attached to the inner walls of the LV and serve to anchor the tethering chords of the mitral valve.

Chapter 3: The EKG Lead System

When visiting a museum, one might view a sculpture while walking past a gallery entrance and moving on. But has there been a true appreciation of the work? To obtain that, the visitor should enter the gallery, walk about the work of art, viewing it from all angles.

The same is true with the heart. It should be examined in its three dimensions. In the introductory remarks, it was noted that an EKG consists of twelve views, each oriented at a different angle. Six of them are called the limb leads and view the heart in the frontal plane of this page, top to bottom, right to left, as with the Vitruvian Man.

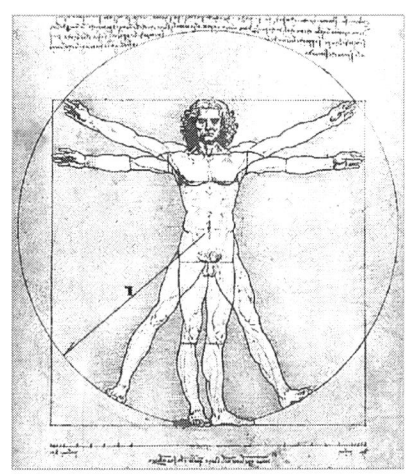

Fig. 6. The Vitruvian Man

The remaining six are called the precordial or V leads (for either ventral or voltage) which eye events as if looking front to back, straight through the page as in the case of Saint Sebastian and the arrows or darts aimed at a bullseye board.

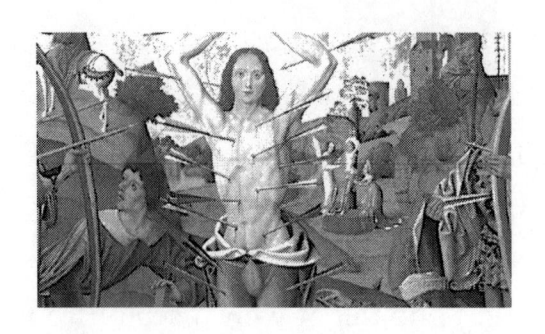

Fig. 7. St. Sebastian

Dr. Willem Einthoven was the Dutch physician and physiologist who pioneered the development of electrocardiography in 1903 and won the Nobel Prize for his work in 1924. His original machine is pictured, Fig. 8. It is amazing that in current times a person can record a very decent one lead trace by placing finger tips on two small metal contacts connected to the app of a mobile device. He was able to record three leads with this apparatus but the technology evolved to allow twelve.

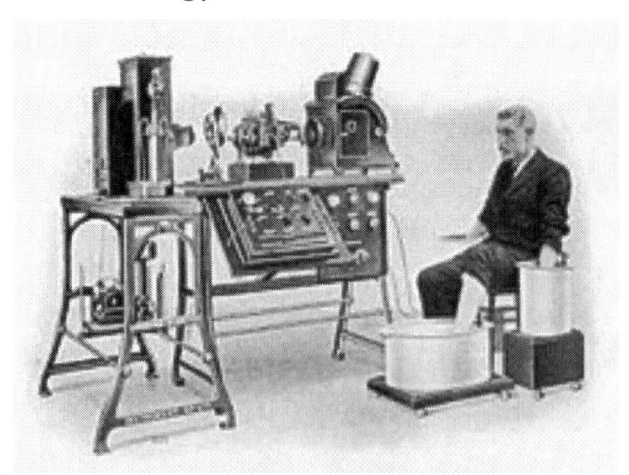

Fig. 8. Dr. Willem Einthoven

Dr. Einthoven began with a triangle, defined by the patient's extremities. First note that in the historic picture he has all limbs, except his right leg, in water containers to assist conductivity. This leg is the equivalent of a ground wire. The three immersed extremities are electrode contact points forming Einthoven's Triangle, defined by the two arms and the left leg. Refer to the drawing below, fig. 9.

By attaching electrode cable tips on the right shoulder and left shoulder, an antenna is created, running horizontally across the heart. This will pick up the signals travelling through the heart (as do all twelve leads) to create an EKG complex. This particular antenna has been given the name limb lead I and is assigned an axis of 0 degrees. Connecting the right shoulder and the left leg creates limb lead II, heading down and to the patient's left. It is located 60 degrees clockwise from lead I (the triangle is assumed to be equilateral). Connecting the left shoulder and the leg defines limb lead III, at 120 degrees pointing down and to the right, relative to the heart.

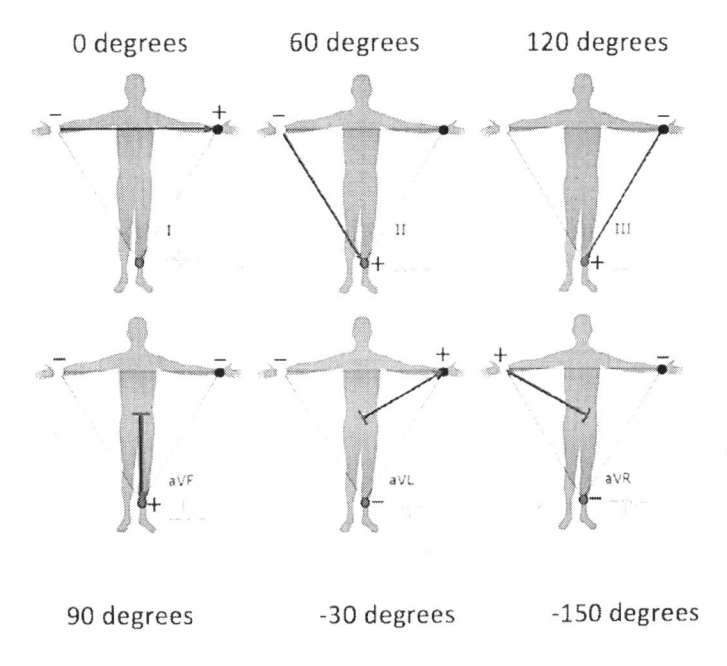

Fig. 9. The six limb leads

Hence there are three leads, each oriented at a different angle from which the same signal is recorded. The signal, leaving the heart on a specific path will have a different appearance in each.

Think of an eyeball at the end of each lead, staring at a statue from its own point of orientation. These three are called *bipolar* leads because *both* ends of each lead are attached to a limb. Note which ends are considered the (+) poles. The importance of knowing this will be discussed soon.

Dr. Einthoven's work led to the development of three more limb leads called aVR, aVL and aVF, for right, left and feet respectively. They provide three more eyeballs at three new viewing angles in the frontal plane. Here, one cable goes from the machine to the right shoulder, one to the left shoulder and one to the left leg. Since there is only *one* contact point on the body for each, these are called *unipolar* leads. If the bipolar leads form a triangle, the unipolar leads form a capital letter Y, superimposed on the triangle, bisecting each 60-degree angle. Again, refer to fig. 9. Lead I is home base: axis designation rotates clockwise to +180 degrees or counterclockwise to -180 degrees (the two points meet at the 9:00 position). Therefore, aVR has an axis of -150 degrees, aVL is at -30 (both counterclockwise from lead I) and aVF is at 90 degrees (clockwise).

The precordial (or V) leads are another six *unipolar* leads that stare inward toward the patient, in an arc across the chest, seeing signal emitted toward them. V lead positioning begins at the fourth right intercostal space on the right side of the sternum and progresses along the curve of the ribs to the fifth intercostal space at the anterior axillary line. They are not assigned angles. Superimposing the six limb leads and the six precordial leads, the illustration below, Fig. 10, nicely demonstrates the entire twelve lead EKG electrode system. Note the heart acts as a central hub and there is a heavy emphasis on the patient's left lower chest quadrant. This is because leads here overlie the left ventricle, the largest source of signal due to its mass. It is critical to remember the lead orientations and the assigned angles (which, to repeat, apply *only* to the six limb leads, not to the V leads).

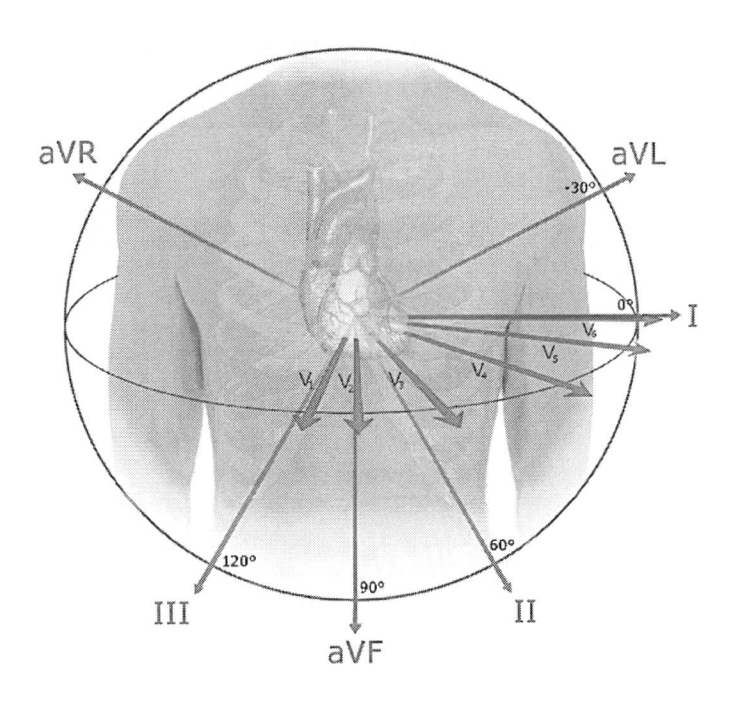

Fig. 10. The 12 lead system

There is a shorthand called "clustering". It is based on the fact that certain leads are neighbors which, together, get similar but not identical views of the heart. For instance, leads II, III and aVF "stare" at the bottom of the heart and for that reason are called the inferior leads. The inferior wall is fed by the right coronary artery in about 90% of the population, termed "right dominant". The remaining 10% are "left dominant" where a large circumflex feeds the inferior wall, a normal variant. Therefore, right coronary/inferior wall ischemia or scar is usually best appreciated in leads II, III and aVF. Leads V1, V2, V3 and V4 are the anterior leads because they are positioned over the anterior wall of the heart and reflect left anterior descending artery/anterior wall events. Leads I, L, V5 and V6 are the lateral leads, all facing the left lateral chest, and roughly report on the circumflex artery. There are further subgroupings of leads. Leads aVR, V1 and V2 are the right sided leads. While V2 is to the left of the sternum, the heart's rotation to the left places that lead over the right ventricle (recall the hand exercise). Leads V3, V4, II, III and aVF are in a central position, lead II being an "honorary" left-of-midline lead and lead III right-of-midline. This will be further discussed when the generation of a normal QRS is considered.

Chapter 4: Factors Influencing Wave Morphology

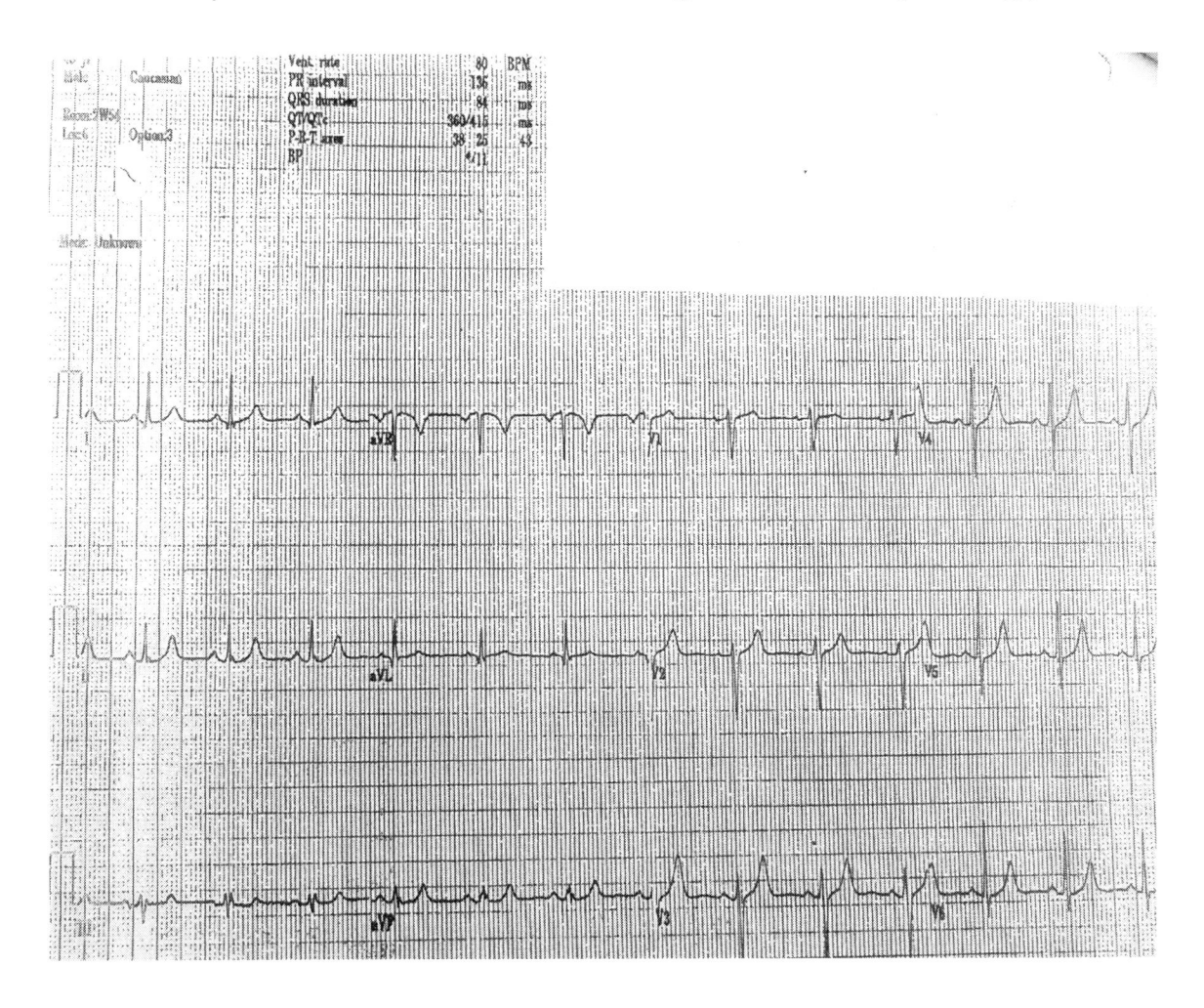

Fig. 11. Normal EKG

A normal 12 lead EKG appears above, Fig. 11. It is recorded left to right, three vertical leads at a time (I, II, III then aVR, aVL, aVF, then V1, V2, V3 and finally V4, V5, V6). Complexes in the same column represent the same heart beat. The smallest boxes are 1mm x 1mm in size. Larger boxes are outlined more boldly, measuring 5 x 5 mm. The paper moves at 25 mm/sec, each mm representing 40 msec of time on the X axis. Vertically, on the Y axis, each 10 mm represents 1.0 mV of amplitude, an indication of chamber muscle mass. A monolith 5 mm wide and 10 mm tall is a shorthand, appearing on the left side of the trace, indicating these scales.

Each wave (P, QRS, T) is described as having *polarity and amplitude*. Polarity refers to direction such as pointing up, down or mixed. Amplitude refers to the degree of height or depth. Three factors determine these features:

-The angle at which a current approaches the "eye" (positive pole) of a specific lead. The eye is always the end where the tip of each arrow is located on fig. 10.

-The mass of the cardiac structure generating the signal.

-The distance the structure is from the recording leads.

The first is the most involved with respect to explanation. Beginning simply, if a signal is headed directly toward a lead's "eye", it registers as an upward deflection. See lead I on the trace above. If headed directly away it will be a negative deflection. See lead aVR. If it runs perpendicular to a lead, it will be *isoelectric* which means flat line or, more usually, as high up as it is deep down. See lead V4.

The appearance of the P wave can be explained by this concept. In order to understand this, you will see how important it is for you to have become familiar with almost everything that has been written so far about gross anatomy, positioning of the heart and conduction system as well as lead orientation. While a signal travels in three dimensions like a cone of light radiating outward from a flashlight, its basic direction –where it starts to where it ends- is represented by a vector. The vector is drawn as a straight arrow representing the center of the beam. In the case of a P wave, the flashlight is pointing down from the SA node to the AV node. Were the anatomical picture of the heart on a map, the P wave signal would travel in a northwest to southeast direction. Think of the trip as from **S**eattle (**S**A node) to **A**tlanta (**A**V node). An airliner is the vector. On radar, the flight path of the P wave will be headed almost exactly towards the positive end of limb lead II, given the orientation the lead was assigned by Einthoven. The wave is therefore an upward deflection in this lead. Conversely, it travels directly away from lead aVR and registers as a negative deflection. *The same event has two opposite appearances and it is all determined by chamber positions, direction of current flow and lead angles.* It is worth mentioning now that the P wave is a small one because of little muscle mass and that the left atrium has very little impact because of it's far distance from the chest wall (signal decays by distance squared).

The QRS is more problematic because it has multiple waves but they do sum up and give an average direction called the *main QRS axis*. Let's discuss the nomenclature of different waves before we proceed further.

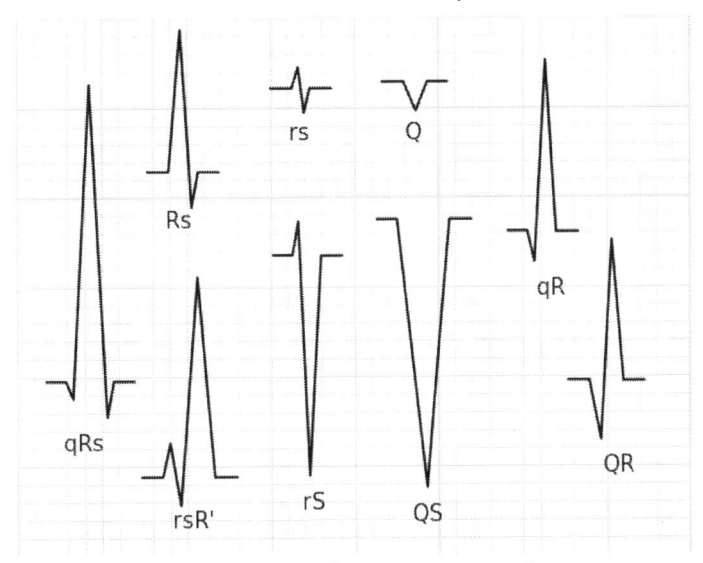

Fig. 12. Waveform nomenclature

An R wave is an upward spike. **R** is on the **R**ise. Q waves and S waves both point down; but a Q wave is distinct as being the first event in the complex (In Great Britain the **Q**ueen is at the head of the royal family; her **S**uccessors are somewhere down the line). An S wave always has an R wave before it.

If there are two upward spikes, the first is R, the second is R-prime (R'). In the diagram, many possibilities are shown. The wave of greatest height can be capitalized. If a wave is only down it is called "Q" or "QS" because the deflection is both first and last.

We use the phrase "R to S ratio" to describe qualitatively the height of the R wave relative to the depth of its own S wave in a QRS complex. Picture a generic lead 1: If a signal's vector points to it, the recorded QRS complex is largely R wave, maybe a tiny S wave; R>S. If it points directly opposite, the complex appears as a tiny R wave and a large S wave; R<S. If the signal is perpendicular, the complex in lead I is isoelectric where R up equals S down in amplitude; R=S. There are intermediary ratios (the degree up relative to the degree down) as one goes from mostly R to mostly S. This is demonstrated by looking at the progression of V leads on the normal EKG in figure 11. See how, in any one lead, an R wave grows proportionally higher *relative to its own* shrinking S. Think of the phases of the moon gradually going from new to crescent to half to gibbous to new over the lunar cycle: the ratio of amount of dark surface (S) to amount of lit surface (R) gradually changes from all dark to all light.

An alternate explanation can be made by visualizing a gas gauge in a car, Fig. 13.

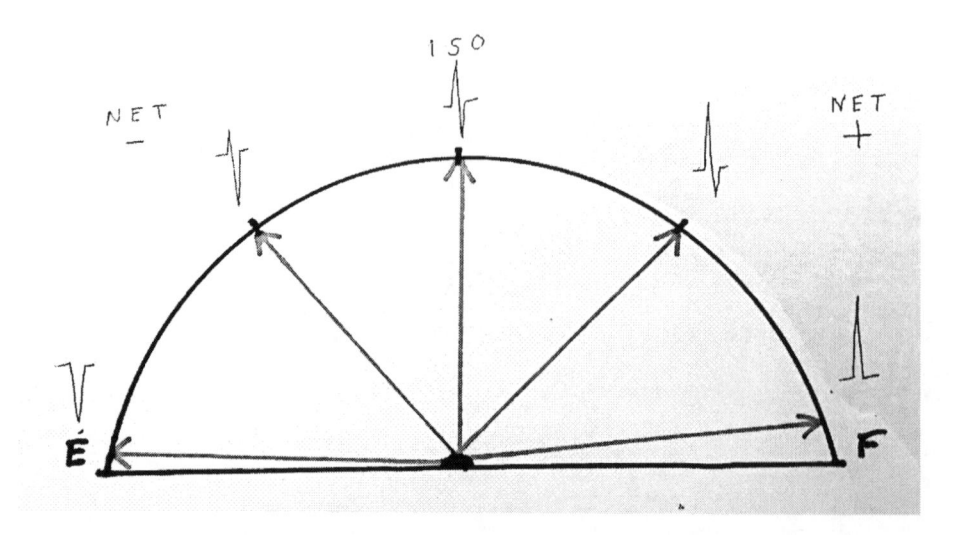

Lead I is the flat linear base. "Full" is its positive pole. The arrows represent a vector at different angles of approach. R wave height represents the amount of gas; S wave depth represents the amount of tank drainage. Starting with a full tank, the needle/vector points directly to full, where the eye of lead I is located, so the QRS is all R wave up as the lead records it. This is an axis of 0 degrees. As the tank drains and the needle moves, the tank has less gas (so R amplitude shrinks) and is of course emptier (so S grows deeper). As long as the tank is more than half full, R will be taller than S is deep (R>S). This is called "net positive". When half a tank is reached, full equals empty, R=S, and the QRS is isoelectric. The QRS axis here is 90 degrees. As soon as the needle sweeps past the halfway mark at 90 degrees, the tank is always more empty than full so R<S, a state called "net negative". At empty, 180 degrees away from tip, the QRS is all S wave.

The bottom line: If a given lead records a net positive QRS, the main axis is aimed somewhere within 90 degrees of the lead, <u>clockwise or counterclockwise</u>. If a lead records a net negative QRS, the main axis is directed more than 90 degrees away, also clockwise or counterclockwise.

Why is so much attention paid to the main QRS axis? There is a range that is considered normal. If the axis falls outside of that range, it may indicate incorrect activation through one of the two trunks constituting the left bundle branch. The trunks are the left anterior and left posterior fascicles. Failure to activate a fascicle can cause a "hemi block" and contribute to serious bradycardia. Left axis may indicate an anterior hemi block and right axis may mean a posterior hemi block. Details will follow in Chapter 9.

What follows is a definition of each type of axis, of which there are four. Consider fig.14. On the clock, 0 degrees begins with lead I at 3:00. Clockwise, axis is progressively more positive until 9:00 (180 degrees).

Counterclockwise from lead I, axis is progressively more negative, again until 9:00 is reached where -180 degrees meets +180 degrees.

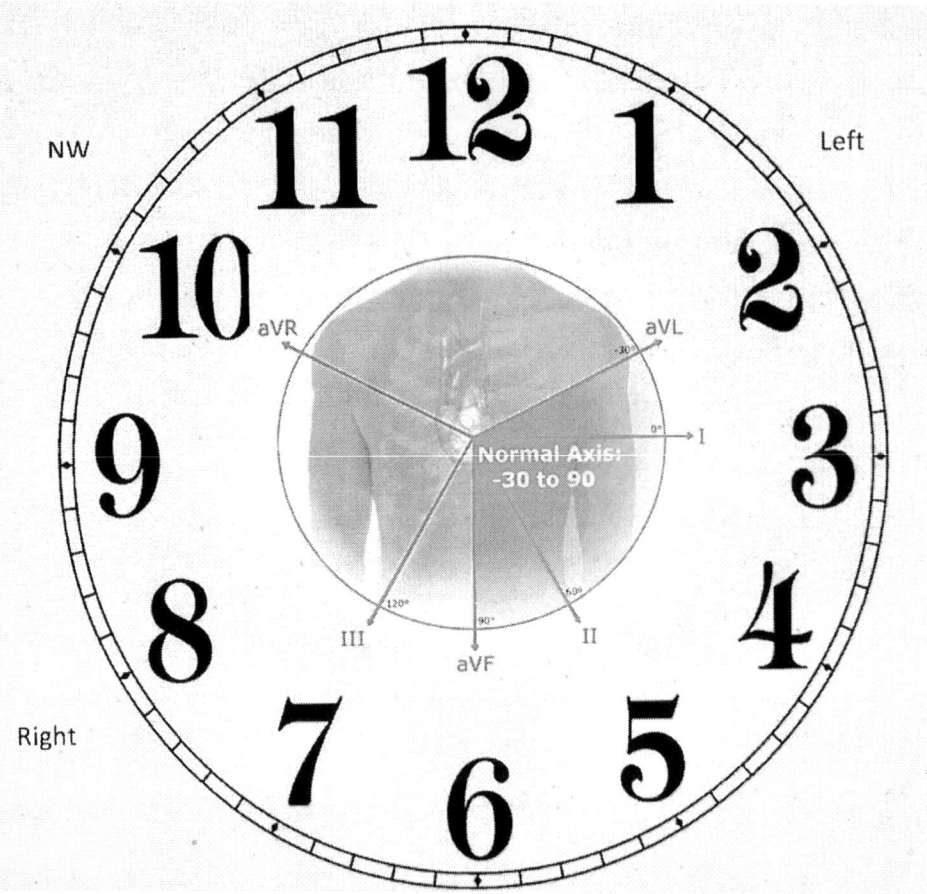

Fig. 14. QRS axis range

A normal main QRS axis is -30 degrees to +90 degrees. This corresponds to 2:00 to 6:00. If the main axis points between -30 degrees and -90 degrees (2:00 back to 12:00) the axis is called "Left". An axis between +90 and +180 degrees (6:00 to 9:00) is "Right". Between 180 and -90 degrees (9:00 to 12:00), the axis is called "Northwest", "Extreme" or "Indeterminate". A quick way of approximating an axis is to find the limb lead that appears most isoelectric. Remember that *only* limb leads are assigned angles. If you refer to the full EKG at the start of this section, you will see limb lead III is most isoelectric. Lead III sits at +120 degrees (7:00) so the main QRS axis is

24

about 90 degrees away (the definition of isoelectric). But which way should we rotate from 120 degrees? Use the clock to assist you. If we move 90 degrees clockwise and find we are at -150 degrees (10:00). If in fact our main QRS axis pointed to this position, lead aVR would be very upright and limb lead I would be very negative. Since neither is so, we move 90 degrees counterclockwise from lead III's position at +120 degrees. We find ourselves at +30 degrees (4:00). This is between lead I at 0 degrees and lead II at 60 degrees and indeed we must be headed in both of their directions because both I and II are very positive. While not easy to read, the computer data panel at the top left of the twelve lead trace calculates the axis as 25 degrees, close to our estimate.

If you practice with an image of the lead system in front of you, a shortcut will be evident revealing whether axis is in normal, left deviated, right deviated or in northwest territory The method uses limb leads I and II because each is 90 degrees away from an abnormal axis. Elsewhere, you may read of other methods to approximate axis; the following one has proven useful in my experience and is based on these facts:

- If lead I records a net positive QRS, axis lies within 90 degrees of the lead's home base at 0 degrees. This can be in either direction: between 12:00 and 6:00 (on the right side of the clock face). If the QRS is net negative, the vector points more than 90 degrees away in either direction, falling between 6:00 and 12:00 (on the left side).

-In similar fashion, if lead II shows a net positive QRS, the vector points between 2:00 and 8:00 on the near side of the clock. If net negative, the vector points between 8:00 and 2:00 on the opposite side.

-Given the above two relationships, determine which half of the clock is appropriate for each lead. Imagine each zone is covered with half of a paper plate. The main QRS axis will lie where the two zones overlap.

Once you are convinced of this, you will see that:

-If **lead I is positive and II is positive**, the axis is **normal** because there is overlap between 2:00 and 6:00, representing -30 to +90 degrees.

-If **lead I is positive and lead II is negative**, there is **left axis** deviation, with the overlap zone between -30 to -90 degrees.

-If **lead I is negative and lead II is positive**, there is **right axis** deviation, since overlap is between +90 and +150 degrees.

-**If both are negative**, the axis is **NW or extreme right.**

There are several exceptions when a right or left axis does not mean a posterior or anterior hemi block, respectively. For instance, a young, tall, thin person with a low lying diaphragm often has a very vertically orientated heart, "dangling" down from the aorta (the word aorta is derived from the Greek for lifter or handle). The axis may appear rightward. Obese people with abdominal fat can have a high lying diaphragm, especially when supine, pushing the cardiac apex up and to the left axis zone. The same can occur with left ventricular hypertrophy because the mass draws current to this zone.

Speaking of left ventricular hypertrophy, we now switch gears. This entire chapter deals with factors that affect the EKG wave morphology and polarity has been addressed. Next is the discussion on amplitude, referring to the height or depth of waves. One factor influencing amplitude is muscle mass. The other is a structure's distance from the chest.

Any cardiac chamber can be enlarged, sometimes from genetic abnormalities, more often from acquired disease. Either atrium can dilate when its associated ventricle is stressed or when there are valve disorders interfering with plumbing. A tight valve (stenotic) blocks drainage; a leaky valve (regurgitant) squirts extra volume backward inappropriately. The right ventricle can enlarge, usually from lung disease which raises the pressure and resistance against which the RV must pump. Left ventricular hypertrophy (LVH) or dilatation (which also increases muscle mass) is usually a result of hypertension, valve disease, ischemic disease, myocarditis, alcohol or congenital hypertrophic cardiomyopathy. Any enlarged chamber sends out a stronger than usual signal in millivolts. Revealing patterns will be discussed as related topics arise.

Amplitude is also affected by distance. Electromagnetic signal strength decays by distance squared (Fig. 15).

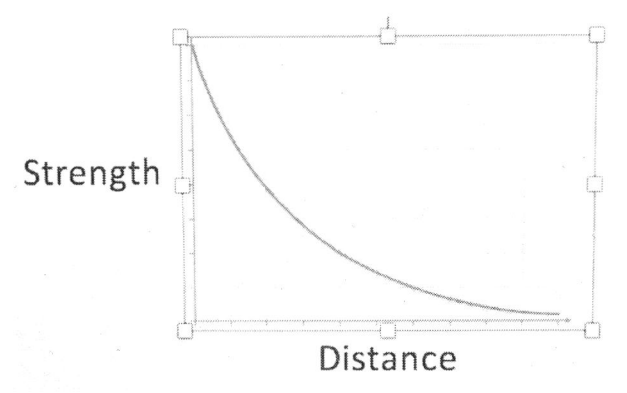

Therefore, a normal left atrium, which is very posteriorly oriented in the chest, has very little influence on a P wave. When enlarged, it has a stronger signal that might override the distance factor as will be seen in the section on P wave morphology. A patient with emphysema might have a hyper inflated, barrel-shaped chest which leaves the heart further from the thoracic wall, "cushioned" by over expanded lungs, resulting in low amplitude signals. Thin patients with little intervening body fat can have tall voltage. In fact, many tall, slender teens are mistakenly diagnosed with left ventricular hypertrophy when none is present. This emphasizes the need to check patient data and clinical indication on an EKG request when interpreting the study.

Chapter 5: The P Wave

As previously discussed, the P wave represents atrial muscular activation, triggered by the repetitive discharge of the sinus node. Fibers run through the RA with branches extending toward the LA, all of which converge at the AV node. The direction of the vector runs from the 10:00 to the 4:00 positions. The tip of lead II is close to being in line with the vector and is best suited to recording a normal P wave as an upright deflection, about 2mm tall. Lead aVR sees the P heading away from it; it is inverted.

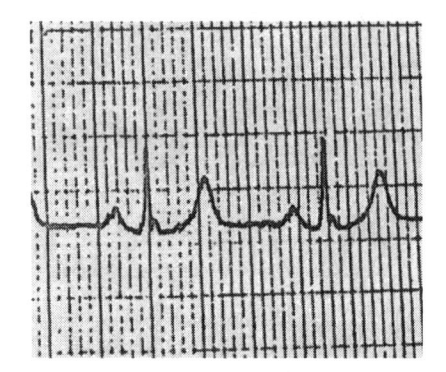

Fig 16. P, upright in lead II

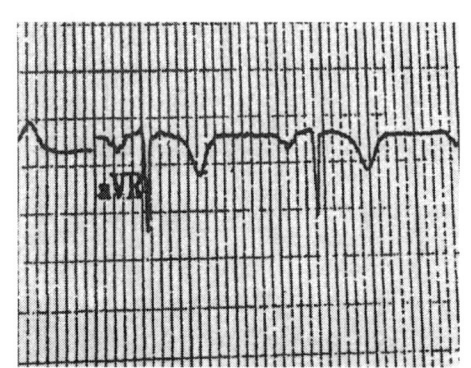

Fig. 17. P, inverted in aVR

The clear appearance of a normal P wave is the reason lead II is called the rhythm strip.

P waves have three obligations: to show up, to be the correct shape and size (amplitude) and to point in the correct direction (polarity). If not present, normal sinus rhythm is absent. If shape or size is incorrect, the RA or LA may be enlarged. If its direction is abnormal, an alternate site in either atrium is the focus of the beat's origin, a phenomenon called ectopy. Examples now follow.

Pressure or volume overload on the right heart, such as that caused by pulmonary hypertension or tricuspid or pulmonic valve disorders, may cause the RA to dilate. With dilatation thickness may remain the same but overall muscle mass is increased. This affects the amplitude of the atrial signal which appears as an unusually tall P wave in lead II. Since direction is the same, from SA node to AV node, this tall P remains upright in that lead. This phenomenon is called "P Pulmonale", P indicating the atrial event and pulmonale indicating the right side of the heart.

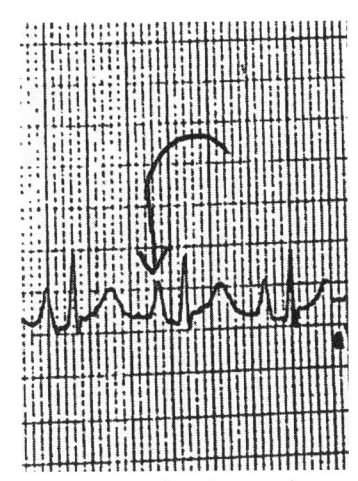

Fig. 18. Peaked P pulmonale

What is "too tall"? The answer is 3 mm on an EKG recorded with standard calibration of 10 mm/mV. This is a good time to discuss interval dimensions in general. Answering a quiz on height or length of many EKG intervals is equivalent to being up at bat in a baseball game: you get three strikes before you're out. It's a good idea to answer 3 or 5 or 1 mm to insure a base hit. For instance, a normal P wave is less than 3 mm high or wide, a normal PR interval is between 3 and 5 mm wide, a normal QRS is less than 3 mm wide, significant ST depression or elevation, indicators of ischemia to be discussed, is more than 1mm. Each will be elaborated upon as we proceed.

Left atrial enlargement can also occur, caused by left sided pressure or volume overload lesions that mirror those affecting the right heart.

Remember that a normal LA signal is negligible due to distance from the front of the chest. When the chamber is enlarged it creates a larger signal, now recordable, but it is still blunted by distance and will have less amplitude than that seen with right atrial enlargement.

To better understand the appearance of LA enlargement, one must think in three dimensions. The RA's contribution to the P wave is evident on all six precordial leads, usually as an upward deflection as seen in the above picture of a normal P in lead II. Returning to an analogy, think of a flashlight sitting in the RA sending out a cone of light along the heart's axis: from 10:00 to 4:00 on a clock face, northwest to southeast, with the end pointing outward. The entire left lower chest, where most of the V leads reside, see some degree of light and record an upward P. Sometimes V1 is too far to the right relative to the heart's orientation and "is in the dark" in which case its P is inverted.

With respect to the LA's contribution, a beam is aimed at the left side of the chest (see the position of Bachmann's Bundle on the drawing of the conduction system, fig. 4). The left lateral V leads are best positioned to see the cone of light heading toward them but V1, positioned on the right side of the chest, sees it heading away.

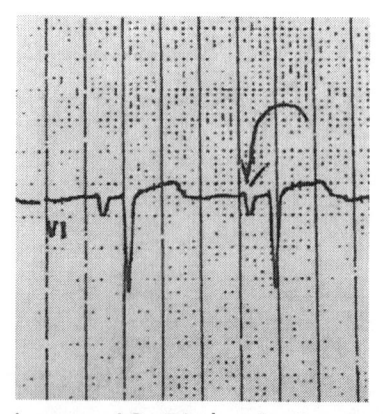

Image 19. Biphasic P wave

Therefore V1 may have an initial positive wave from the RA followed by a terminal negative deflection due to the left atrial signal's opposing path. This is called a "biphasic P wave", seen in Fig. 19, labelled with an arrow. If we could record directly from the surface of the left atrium the deflection would be quite large; but by the time it travels from the rear to the front of the chest, where the lead is attached, it only needs to be 1 mm deep to be considered abnormally deep.

A second pattern showing a large LA can be seen in a left sided lead such as V5 or V6; this appears as two serial upward waves (fig, 20), first from the RA and then from the LA. The recording has a rounded letter M shape.

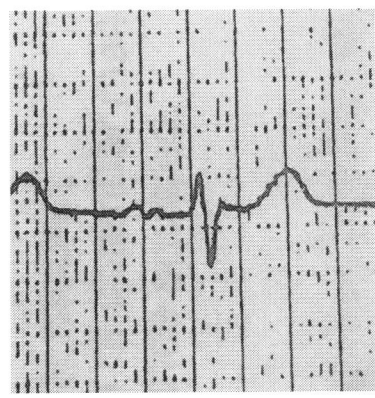

Fig.20. M-shaped P mitrale

This is called P Mitrale (P **P**ulmonale is **P**eaked, P **M**itrale is **M**-shaped). It is 3 or more mm wide reflecting the increased time needed to cross the bulkier LA. Either one of the above two patterns is sufficient to meet criteria for LA enlargement. It is not necessary to have both appear on a single trace.

The next figure (21) helps explain LA enlargement. In one pattern, V1 sees the front arrow (the RA's component of the P wave) radiating out as an upward deflection. It sees the LA's component, indicated by the rear arrow

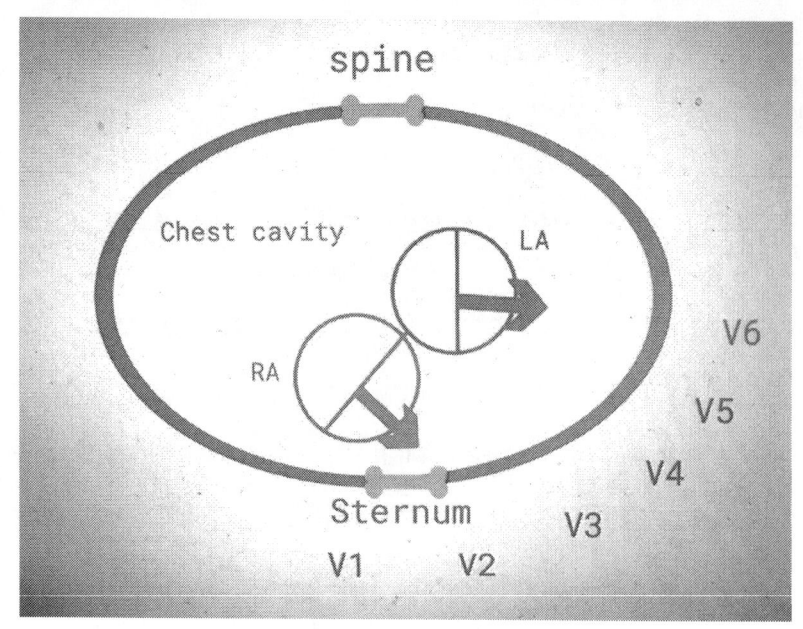

Fig. 21- looking from overhead

heading away from it, as a downward wave. The P wave is biphasic. In the alternate pattern V5 and V6 have the benefit of seeing light radiating from *both* the RA and LA arrow, giving rise to the m-shaped P wave called P-Mitrale.

Chapter 6: The QRS complex

The size of the of the ventricles, their masses and volumes all require a more complicated set of nerve fibers necessary for activation. These include the right bundle branch (RBB) to the RV and the left bundle branch (LBB) to the LV, the latter being larger to meet the demands of the thicker chamber. In fact, the LBB has two trunks called left anterior and left posterior fascicles which are interconnected very well by cross fibers made of myelinated nerve tissue, like rungs between two posts of a ladder. Until later, the two fascicles will be treated as one large trunk. The LBB also supplies the septum with a twig, going left to right, which is the common wall at the midline of the two ventricles. The septum, shared by both, is like a child in the midst of a divorce; the better-endowed parent supplies child support.

Travelling down both bundle branches simultaneously is efficient and rapid because they are myelinated nerves. Current can be carried by myocardial tissue but myocardial cells are not myelinated so current runs through more slowly. Think of the RBB and LBB as two ski slopes descending Heart Mountain. Normally two skiers begin at a common peak point of origin (the Bundle of His) and simultaneously travel down their respective slopes, each covering his or her side of the mountain. If for some reason a slope is not accessible – for example, this is what happens if a bundle branch block is present- a skier will first speed down the healthy side and then slowly travel cross country and uphill over the deficient side, made up of non-myelinated, slowly conducting muscle tissue. This will widen a QRS but insures that, under all circumstances, the whole heart is electrically activated.

There are several conditions when a current gets off-track and must travel across myocardium. As mentioned, a bundle branch block is one. So are beats that are initiated by deep ventricular tissue (such as premature ventricular contractions). A third example is abnormal conduction due to re-routing, as in Wolf-Parkinson-White Syndrome. These will be covered later. For now, a description of a normal QRS will be explained with the help of the next diagram.

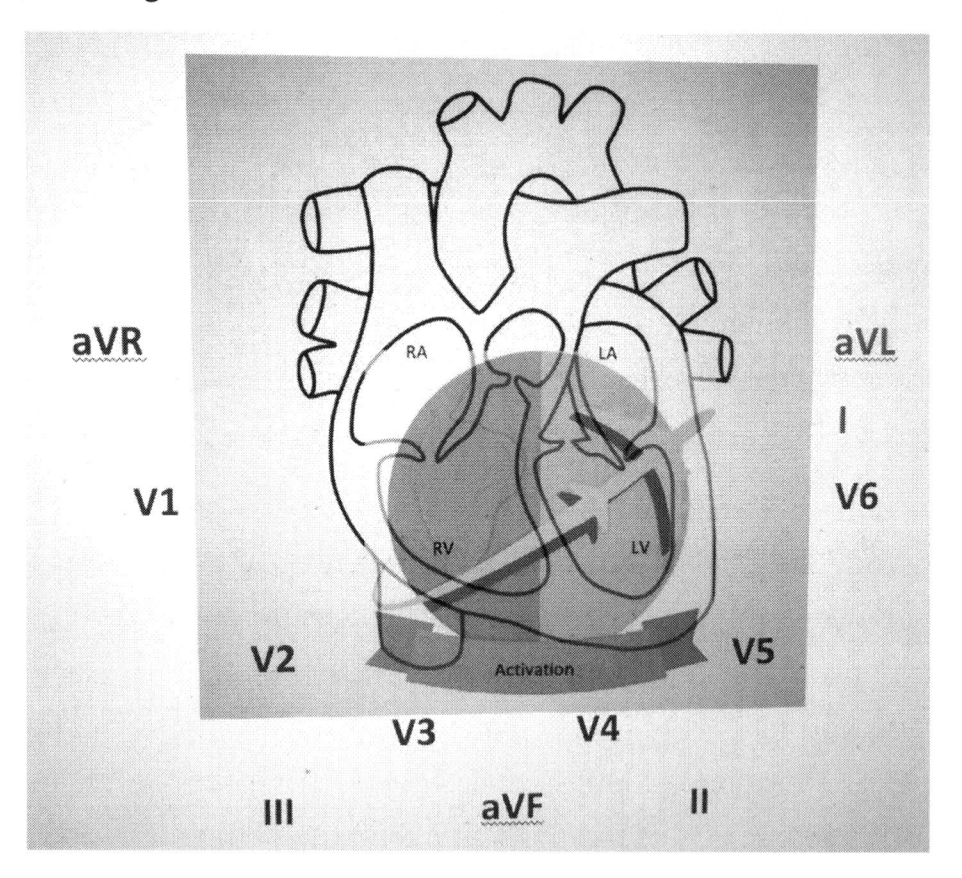

Fig. 22, Ventricular activation

First, the grand design (then the details): Right sided leads (aVR, V1 and V2) see low amplitude R waves from low mass right heart signal aimed toward them, and deep S waves from high mass left heart signal heading away from them. They are net negative. Reciprocally, the left sided leads (I, aVL, V5 and V6) may see tiny Q waves from the distant right heart signal heading away, but mostly high R waves from the left heart signal heading towards them (they are net positive). Central leads (V3, V4, II, III and aVF) transition from net negative to isoelectric to net positive.

Now for the details: After activating the atria and briefly stalling in the AV node, the current passes through the Bundle of His. Then it descends the RBB through the RV, aiming down and to the patient's right. It also enters the LBB where, early on, the twig that feeds the septum also directs current from left to right as well as downward through that mid wall. Together, the signals radiate out from the edge of the right heart in the region of the narrow tail of the jet's contrail, aiming toward V1 and V2. These leads record a small R wave, small because the RV and septum are not as massive as the LV. Lead aVR is too far in the upper right to register this. In theory, the far left sided leads see these rightward directed signals and would be expected to register a Q wave but their distance away and the small mass responsible for the current often make this deflection inherently small and negligible.

Then the jet turns and begins its sweep across the front of the globe toward the left side of the chest. This represents the sequence of activation which covers the anterior, inferior and apical walls of the heart, both west to east and south to north, pretty much what we see head-on. The mid positioned leads, such as V3, V4, and the inferior leads, are the first ones in this part of the path and see increasingly greater signal, with taller R waves the further to the left the leads are positioned. This is because they are getting closer to the main QRS axis. By this time in the sequence, V4 and lead II should be net positive.

At the same time, the right sided leads see the strong current building to the left and this results in deep S waves developing in their recordings, so they become net negative.

The jet continues, passing over the left lateral side of the globe, maximizing R waves in the left sided leads, V5, V6, lead I and aVL because they are often in the direct path of a normally angled main QRS axis, the strongest part of the signal. S waves get still deeper in right sided leads.

Finally, as the jet curves around to the back of the globe, its turn directs it to the patient's right again, covering the high posterior wall of the LV, the last zone to be activated, so the left sided leads may end with a terminal S wave. That same rightward direction of the flight may even cause a second small R wave to appear in V1, called R prime. This last signal is usually small or not even recorded, since it arises from far back, behind the heart.

Again, summing this up, right sided leads are net negative, left sided leads are net positive and mid positioned leads are in-between. Leads III and V3 are right-central and are usually net negative. Lead II and V4 are left-central and, by this time in the course of things, have usually switched to net positive. For this reason, these are called transitional leads.

Remember the importance of main QRS axis variability. If vertical, as in a young, tall and thin patient, the inferior leads may see the strongest signal and have the most prominent R waves. The axis can be aimed downward so much even V5 and V6 start to lose R wave amplitude. They have "overshot" the main beam. On the other hand, if axis is very leftward, R wave may be of poor amplitude throughout most of the precordial and inferior leads. The beam has shifted too far away from them.

Below is a copy of the normal EKG to demonstrate the *usual* findings.

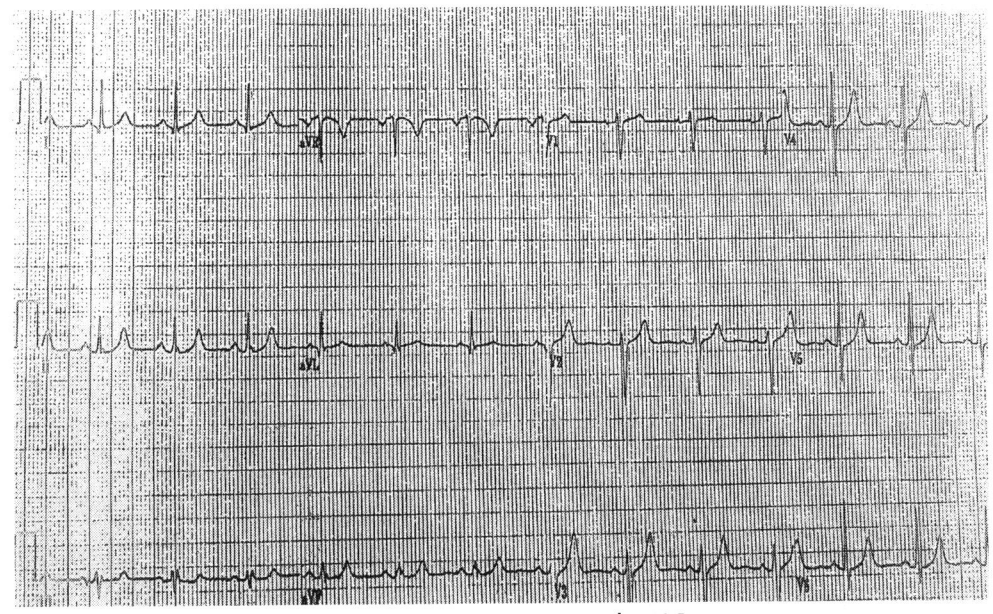

Figure 23. Normal EKG

-Right sided leads aVR, V1 and V2 are net negative.

-Left sided leads I, aVL, V5 and V6 are net positive.

-Right-central leads III and V3 are, or approach, net negative while left-central leads V4 and II are, or approach, net positive. These are the transitional leads.

-Notice the terminal S waves in V5 and V6 from the end of activation which, as described, terminates toward the right to stimulate the high posterior wall of the LV.

-In the V leads, as one progresses to the left (V1 to V6), the R:S ratio should get progressively higher. This is called R wave progression. Failure of the ratio to progress may mean R waves are blunted because underling myocardium has been partially thinned out by scar (scar sends no signal, to be discussed later) or because an axis is very far to the left in which case the V leads are out of range of the strongest part of the signal. Sometimes, in women with large breasts, increased wall thickness from underlying adipose tissue may reduce the entire sizes of V5 and V6, R and S alike, but this is not a problem as long as each R wave is progressively larger than *its own* S wave.

-Finally, from the trace, note that T waves are upward except in aVR. They may or not be inverted in other right sided leads such as V1 and lead III, though this is not demonstrated in Fig. 22. In young people T inversion may extend to V2, a normal variant in these circumstances.

We have seen the abnormalities that can affect P wave morphology. With respect to the QRS, irregularities usually involve amplitude, duration and shape. Higher than expected amplitude may mean ventricular hypertrophy or dilatation.

-Right ventricular hypertrophy (RVH): this is seen with chronic pulmonary hypertension. Acute dilatation may be seen with a massive pulmonary embolus. On occasion, adult survivors of congenital heart disease such as Tetrology of Fallot or longstanding ventricular septal defects may present with evidence of right ventricular overload. If the RV is enlarged its usually small signal becomes larger. This is reflected by unexpectedly large R waves in V1 and V2 which become net positive, sometimes with a "splintering" of the QRS, taking the form of an RSR' due to the increased time it takes for the right-directed current to cross the enlarged chamber.

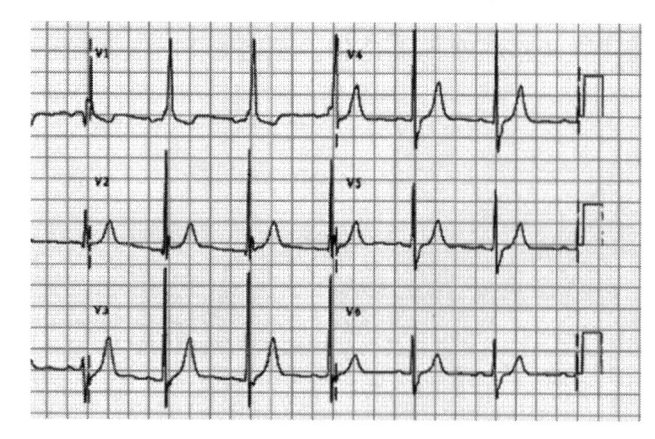

Fig. 24. RVH in the V leads

Left ventricular hypertrophy (LVH) is usually considered present when the depth of the S wave in V1 (reflecting LV forces directed away from that position) plus the height of the R wave in either V5 or V6 (representing the same forces headed towards their position) exceeds 35 mm. An R > 11 mm in lead I or aVL is another sign suggesting LVH. In addition to high voltage on the Y axis, the QRS is sometimes widened on the X axis to 3 mm (120 msec) versus the usual 2 mm (80 msec) due to increased transit time across the more muscular chamber. Often there is abnormal repolarization which takes the form of ST depression and T wave inversion in left sided leads, a term some call "strain pattern", a more preferred name being "associated repolarization abnormalities". These changes have similar appearances to ischemic changes, seen later, but do not represent true ischemia when voltage criteria for LVH are met unless a patient has suggestive signs or symptoms of coronary insufficiency. Also be wary if such changes are new.

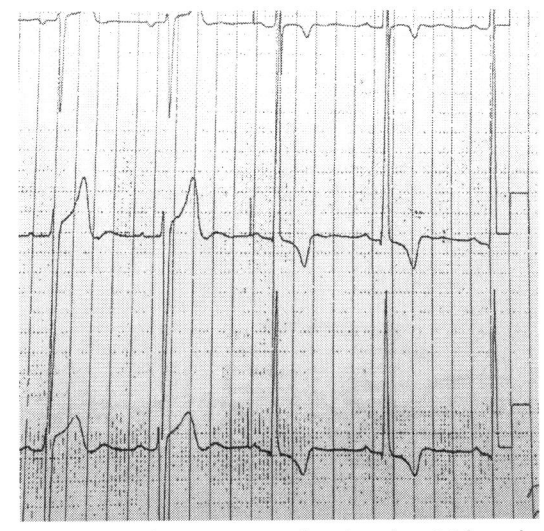

Fig. 25. LV hypertrophy in the V leads

Reference was made to a wider than normal QRS. In the case of LVH, this is called intraventricular conduction delay (IVCD). Other causes, to be seen later, are right bundle branch block (RBBB), left bundle branch block (LBBB), a delta wave from Wolf-Parkinson-White Syndrome (WPW) or a beat originating from either ventricle. As already mentioned, an example of the last is a premature ventricular contraction (PVC). A normal QRS uses both bundle branches and has a duration of about 80 msec (2 mm on standard recording speed). With a bundle branch block, one branch is efficiently used, the other isn't so the QRS lasts 120 msec (3 mm). A beat of ventricular origin starts ectopically in the ventricle, misses both bundle branches, travels through myocardium alone, and lasts at least 160 msec (4 mm).

An IVCD has the appearance of normal QRS complexes on the EKG but the complexes are wider, as if the paper were rubber and slightly stretched side to side. See Fig. 26. Sometimes the QRS may look fragmented. The appearances represent a longer activation time (120 msec), usually due to more muscle mass, but may reflect the effect of medications.

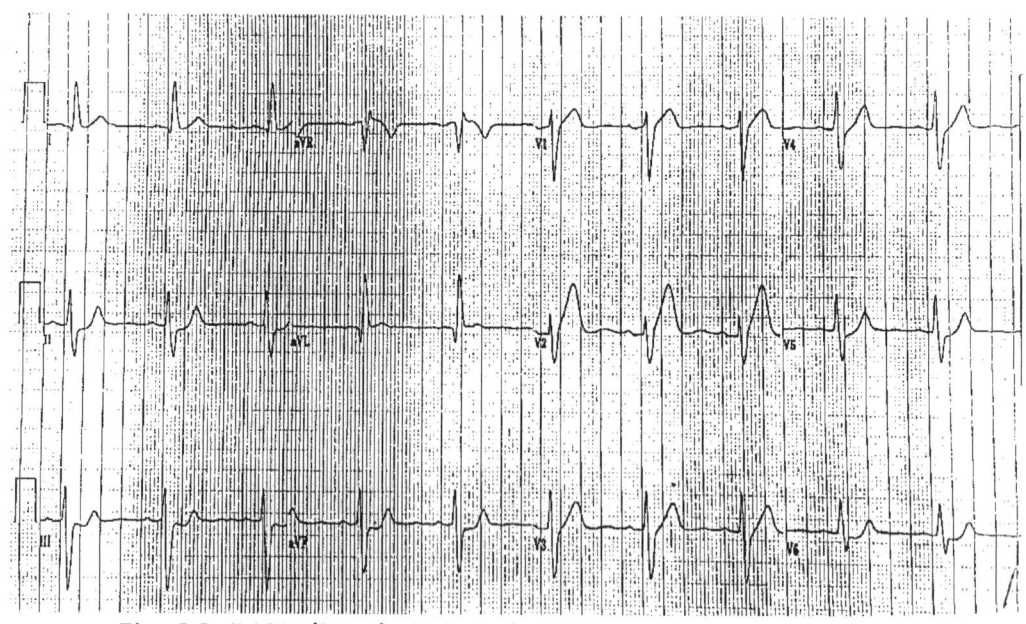

Fig. 26. IVCD (isoelectric in lead II. Axis is -30 degrees)

For example, antiarrhythmic drugs such as quinidine or sotalol are used to suppress abnormally generated rhythms that compete with normal sinus rhythm. These medications act in three ways: 1) by an anesthetic-like effect, suppressing the random "sparking" called automaticity, a premature ventricular contraction (PVC) for example, 2) by slowing conduction time so that an abnormal focus is sluggish in its propagation and less likely to compete with normal tissue, and 3) by prolonging recovery time, or refractory period, so that an abnormal focus cannot regenerate itself, taking longer to recuperate from its last cycle, thus giving normal rhythm more time to intervene first. But, like chemotherapy, these medications may not distinguish health tissue from unhealthy. They may affect a normal QRS and slow its conduction time down, giving rise to the IVCD. Also, some antiarrhythmic medication slow normal sinus node sparking, causing sinus bradycardia. Some lengthen normal recovery, causing a prolonged QT interval, a phenomenon which, as we will see, can backfire and promote fatal rhythm disturbances, such as torsades-de-pointes. Hyperkalemia has a similar effect on prolonging conduction time. Early on, T waves are sharply peaked. Then, as if the P, QRS and T were fashioned out of a cord, increasing K+ levels has the effect of pulling the two ends apart, slowing the rate and slurring and flattening all waves – until it is flat line.

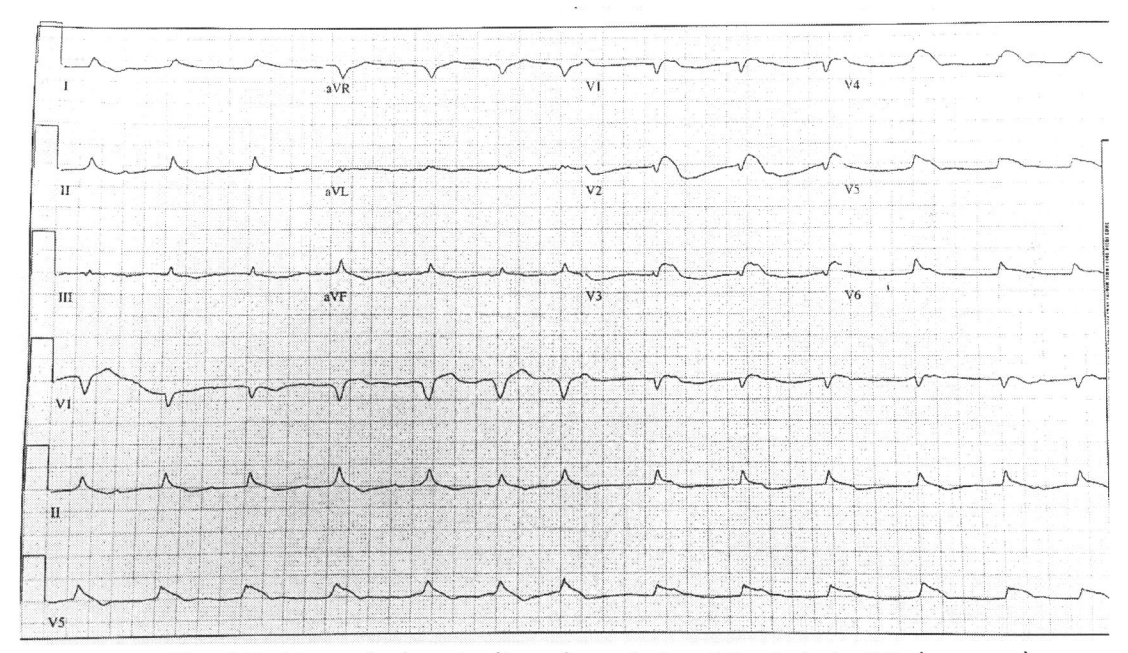

Fig. 27. Hyperkalemia (isoelectric in aVL. Axis is 60 degrees)

Bundle branch blocks widen the QRS. In the presence of a RBBB, there is normal activation of the septum and left ventricle by the left bundle. The initial R wave and terminal S wave in V1 appears the same. However, there is no normal activation of the RV, so after the rapid left sided conduction has occurred, a slow current moves from the left, as with cross country, uphill skiing, toward the right, through the muscle of the RV. Being slow (wide), late (at end of complex) and aimed at V1 (upright), there is a terminal, broad R' in that lead. At this time, the left side is silent electrically so the R' in the RV, as the only "voice", is tall in closely adjacent V1.

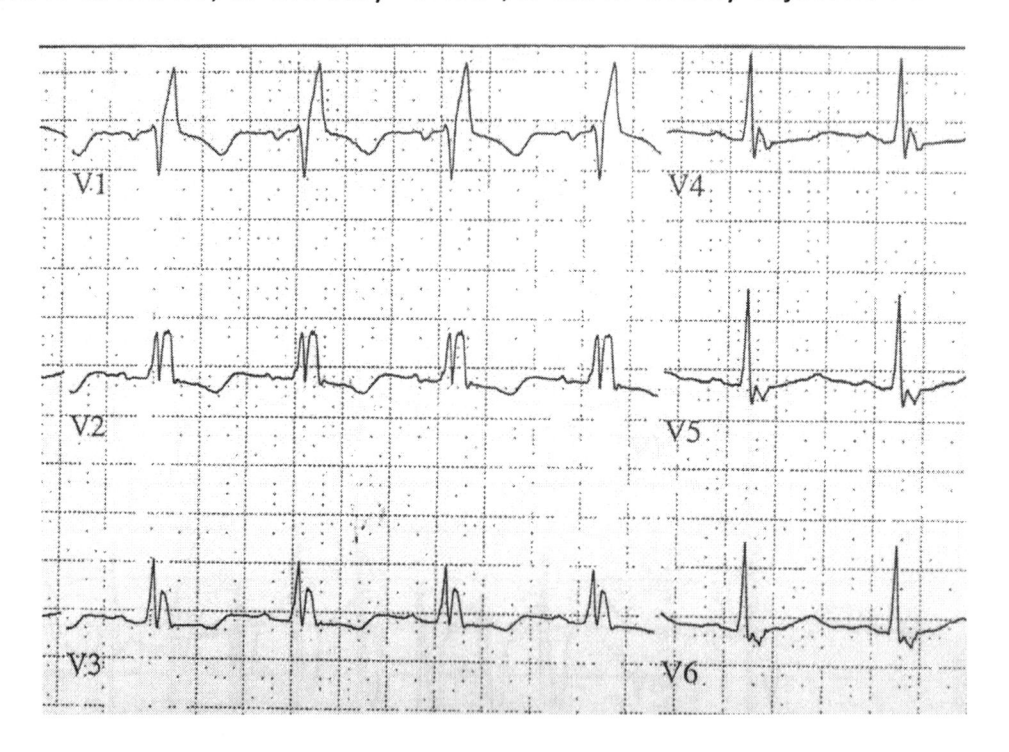

Fig. 28. RBBB in V leads

Reciprocally, as viewed from a left sided lead, say aVL, there is a broad terminal S wave, reflecting the same late, slow current heading to the RV, away from the left. Recorded from the opposite side of the chest, the pattern in aVL is an inverted copy of the one seen in V1. Due to aVL's far distance from the right heart, its terminal broad S wave is rather shallow compared to the tall R' in V1.

In V1 this pattern of a small R, downward S and late terminal large R' (abbreviated rSR') has been described as an asymmetric set of "rabbit ears." Visually, this may be stretching the analogy a bit but, nonetheless, it helps to remember **RaBB**it ears in V1 indicate RBBB. In image 28 note the rSR' in V1 and broad terminal notched S in V5 and V6.

A LBBB is easier to understand. There is no initial septal activation because that twig arises from the nonfunctioning left bundle branch. The ventricular signal first travels down the right bundle and then slowly crosses the septum and the LV through myocardial tissue, heading to the left, appearing as a deep wide QS trough in V1 or a tall broad R in left sided leads. Often, after crossing the septum, there is a brief backtracking, left to right, to "retrieve" the septum missed by the nonfunctioning twig. Then the path

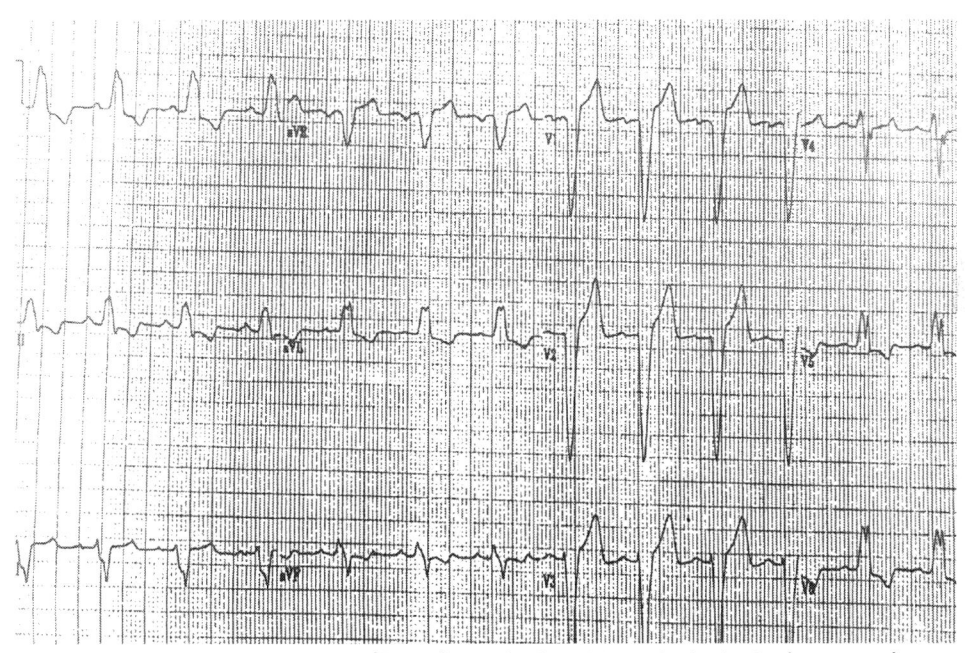

Fig. 29. LBBB (isoelectric in aVF. Axis is 0 degrees)

shifts back to its leftward course, causing a splintering near the QRS peak in the left sided leads There are expected abnormal ST and T waves with a LBBB and they are usually oriented in the opposite direction of the QRS.

In Fig. 29, note the trough in V1, the splintering in V5 and V6 and the orientation of the ST and T waves with both being depressed when QRS is predominantly up and both being elevated when QRS is mostly down.

WPW is an unusual condition, the equivalent of having two AV nodes, the normal one located centrally and the other one, called a bypass tract, located off to the side, left or right. A P wave prefers travelling down the bypass tract because it conducts more rapidly. This results in a short PR interval, less than 3 mm. While this spark has entered a ventricle faster than usual by using the bypass tract, it is far to the side. It must slowly cross ventricular muscle tissue at the start of the QRS in order to get back on track

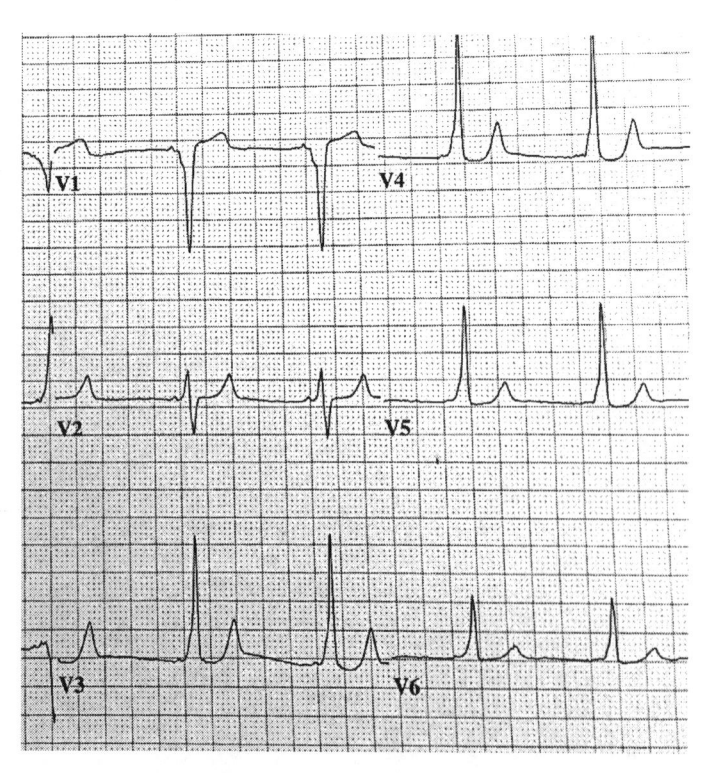

Fig 30. Wolf-Parkinson-White Syndrome

with the normal bundle branches which arise from the Bundle of His (near the central AV node). This initial slow transit is responsible for a slurred delta wave, widening the QRS which is why it is discussed in this section. Remember, a short PR and a delta wave are the hallmarks of WPW.

In fig. 30, these findings are nicely demonstrated in V1 but this lead is not always the best to demonstrate the criteria. The bypass tract can be between RA and RV or between LA and LV, anterior of posterior, so one cannot predict a single specific "go-to" lead to make the diagnosis, versus the **utility of always using V1 to diagnose bundle branch blocks (RBBB - rabbit ears- or LBBB – deep trough)**. In suspected WPW a short PR is the tip off; be sure to check multiple leads for a delta wave.

This is a convenient time to discuss the hemi blocks. Picture the LV as a glass jar. The two branches of the left bundle branch, as stated, are like posts of a ladder with connecting rungs, all composed of rapidly conducting nerve tissue. The ladder sits upright in the LV jar with the posterior fascicle running down the septum medially and the anterior fascicle running down the lateral wall. If there is a left anterior hemi block (LAHB), current runs down the healthy posterior fascicle adjacent to the septum, then slides quickly across the myelinated rungs, laterally and upwards toward the high left side of the heart, to activate the territory which relied on the now-blocked anterior fascicle. This draws the main QRS axis into left deviation territory. Therefore, a main QRS axis more negative than -30 degrees is a clue that a LAHB is present. In the case of a left posterior hemi block (LPHB), which is less frequently seen because this fascicle is thicker and has a better blood supply, current runs down the lateral post of the ladder, then shifts across the rungs down and to the right, yielding an axis greater than +90 degrees, into right deviation territory. There is no widening of the QRS because the connecting branches are made of nerve tissue and there is no need (as there would be with a full bundle branch blocks) to utilize non-myelinated myocardial tissue as a path and no need to slowly cross the septum because all activity is in one chamber, the LV.

Other conditions have been discussed that cause right and left axis deviation (tall thin youths and stout supine patients, respectively) so there are more refined criteria for true hemi blocks. In LAHB, the initial signal in the healthy posterior branch is medially directed toward the right chest giving a Q wave in lead I. At the end of the trip, all is heading leftward, giving a S in lead III. Therefore, a left axis with a QI-SIII pattern is a more precise definition of LAHB. In the case of LPHB, initial forces are aimed laterally to the left (Q in lead III) and then shift heavily to the right at the conclusion (S in lead I). So right axis with QIII-SI is indicative of LPHB.

The following shorthand will be useful when discussing heart block later:

-Unifascicular block means one of three fascicles is not functioning. This could be RBBB (rabbit ears in V1 on the precordial lead side of a 12 lead trace), or LAHB (left axis in the limb lead side), or LPHB (right axis deviation).

-Bifascicular block means two fascicles are diseased. The possible combinations of two out of three include: RBBB + LAHB (rabbit ears in V1 plus left axis in limb leads), RBBB + LPHB (rabbit ears in V1 plus right axis in limb leads) or LBBB alone (deep trough in V1. Axis doesn't count. It is very variable with a LBBB).

-If bifasciular block is present, there is risk the remaining fascicle might falter. This is trifascicular block, leaving no path for a signal to enter the ventricles, risking asystole. Fortunately, as discussed earlier, there is a backup but very slow escape pacemaker that arises from the ventricle called an idioventricular rhythm firing in the 20's or 30's which attempts to sustain life. More will be presented later in Chapter 9.

Chapter 7: Arrhythmias – Part 1, Ectopic Type

The ideal rhythm arises from the sinus node at a rate of 60 to 100 beats per minute in a resting adult. There are simple irregularities in sinus rhythm such as sinus bradycardia (rate below 60 at rest), sinus tachycardia (rate over 100 at rest) and a visible variation in tempo called sinus arrhythmia where the two closest beats on a trace differ from the two furthest by at least one big box (0.2 seconds). An example and further discussion will follow.

Having dispensed with these, all other arrhythmias have one of two mechanisms: ectopic or reentrant. Ectopic rhythms are generated from "renegade" sites firing from a non-sinus site such as myocardial tissue. These are random, irregular and microscopic in origin. They are focal, like the moons of Jupiter. Reentrant rhythms occur when a signal travels in a normal forward, anterograde, direction down some electrical fibers in the heart but abnormally loops upward, retrograde, through other fibers. It then turns back to anterograde, continuing the circuitous route like a merry-go-round or the rings of Saturn. Both ectopic and reentrant rhythms can arise from the supraventricular or ventricular zones.

There are distinctions between the electrical systems in these two regions. "Supraventricular" refers to the sinus node, the atria, the AV node and the Bundle of His. These rely heavily on the right coronary artery for blood supply and are slowed down by increasing vagal tone (progressive sinus bradycardia and progressive prolongation of conduction through the AV node). Assuming no downstream conduction delays, such as a bundle branch block or delta wave, supraventricular QRS complexes are narrow. "Ventricular" refers to the bundle branches, the Purkinje fibers and the ventricular muscle tissue. These are not affected electrically by the vagus nerve and have a greater reliance on the left anterior descending artery because that vessel generally has the most ventricular distribution. A beat of ventricular origin always displays broad QRS complexes. As previously stated, a normal QRS is 2 mm wide because it employs both healthy bundle branches. With a bundle branch block, one bundle is used while slower muscle transmission finishes the cycle; so the QRS is widened, but only to 3 mm. In a beat of ventricular origin, neither bundle branch is used normally; the current runs entirely through muscle and the QRS duration is at least 4 mm wide. Recalling the analogy of Heart Mountain, a ventricular beat is equivalent to a skier beginning to cover the mountain from the bottom; it travels cross country and uphill over both sides.

After describing sinus arrhythmia, ectopic rhythms will be covered followed by reentrant rhythms.

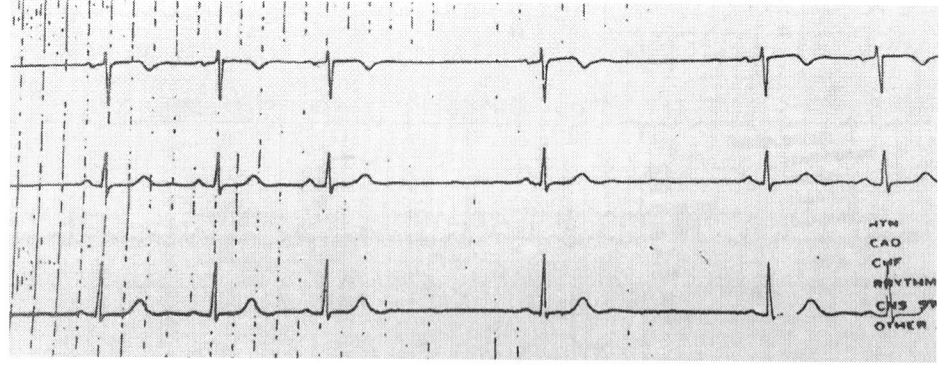

Fig. 31. Sinus arrhythmia

Sinus arrhythmia is not necessarily abnormal. It is usually seen in the pediatric population where it is physiologic. On deep inspiration, blood is sequestered in the expanding lungs. Less returns to the left atrium. In order to maintain cardiac output as volume goes down, heart rate accelerates, mediated by pressure and volume sensors in the circulation which direct vagal tone. Upon exhalation, the lungs are "wrung out" with increased left atrial return. Heart rate declines. As adults we outgrow this sensitive reflex so that a change in heart rate with respiration is minimal unless there is respiratory distress such as with status asthmaticus. When seen in an adult to the degree illustrated in the above sample, there is usually an abnormal cause: rate lowering drugs or age related changes in sinus node function, a form of "sick sinus syndrome". Note that all P waves are identical in any one lead.

As a model for true ectopic rhythms, premature atrial contractions (PAC's) will be presented at length. An abnormal focus fires randomly anywhere in either atrium. Adrenaline, pharmacologic and illicit stimulants, tobacco, alcohol, lung disease and excessive thyroid hormone may cause this. If the focus is far from the sinus node, it traverses the atria in an abnormal path and registers as an abnormally shaped P wave. Consider a source low in the right atrium. The vector travels in the same direction as, say, Texas to New York. It will appear as a P wave inverted in the inferior leads. Occurring prematurely, the stimulus will still attempt to generate a QRS but it will also pass over the sinus node, negating the next expected sinus beat, leading to a larger than expected interval between the premature beat and the next recovered sinus beat, called a compensatory pause. This delay allows the heart a longer diastolic filling time and a greater end diastolic filling volume. Like an overstretched rubber band, the heart has a more pronounced recoil. This is sensed as a "palpitation".

In the illustration, Fig. 32, the arrow points to the early, misshapen P wave. Note the compensatory pause. Sometimes the ectopic source lies close to the sinus node and its P wave is only slightly different from a normal sinus P. Be sure to check all 12 leads to search for a distinct difference no matter how subtle.

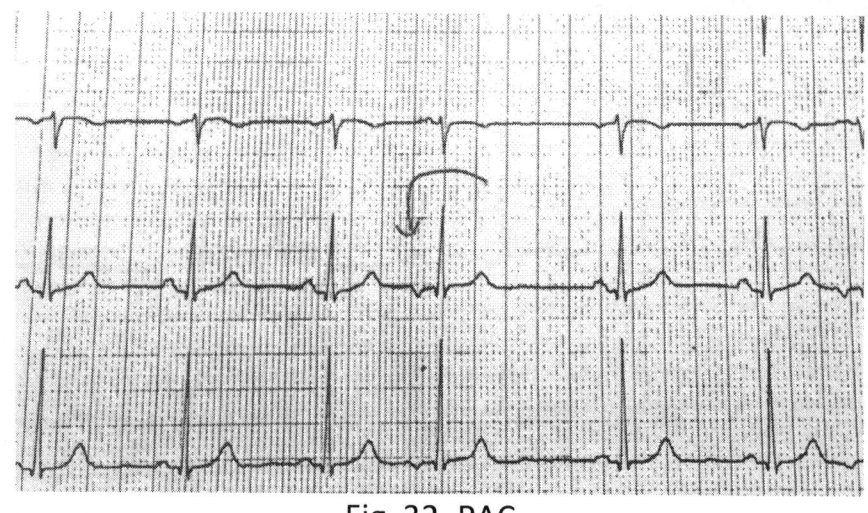

Fig. 32. PAC

In real estate, the mantra is "location, location, location". In electrophysiology, it's "timing, timing, timing". Since a PAC is random it might occur very close to the previous beat's QRS-T complex. Immediately after the earlier normal beat, the heart may still be in its refractory period, the time it takes to reorganize ionic channels so that they are prepared to give an effective subsequent beat. The refractory period varies between the two bundle branches so that one of them might be ready to fire with a repeat early challenge while the other is as yet unable. Therefore, a very early PAC might enter the ventricle and conduct down one branch and not the other, the model for a bundle branch block. This is called a PAC with aberrancy. The phenomenon is termed rate-related aberrancy. Below in Fig. 33 there are two leads: V1 on top, lead II on the bottom. The first arrow points to the premature P. Note it is early and in lead II it is inverted, a clue to abnormal source point. The QRS is identical to its predecessor. The second arrow points to another PAC. Its P wave is earlier than the first, i.e. landing on top of the previous beat's T wave. Here, the ventricle is still partially refractory. The right bundle branch has not yet "recuperated" but the left has, so the QRS has a typical RBBB (rabbit ear) pattern in V1.

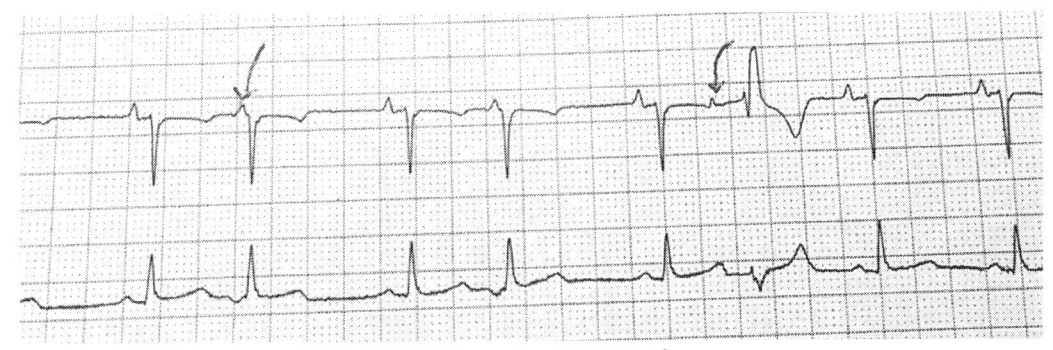

Fig. 33. PAC with RBBB aberrancy

How do we know that this is not a premature <u>ventricular</u> contraction? The answer is that it is preceded by an ectopic P wave, indicating an atrial/supraventricular origin. A PVC has no atrial trigger as shown in this illustration.

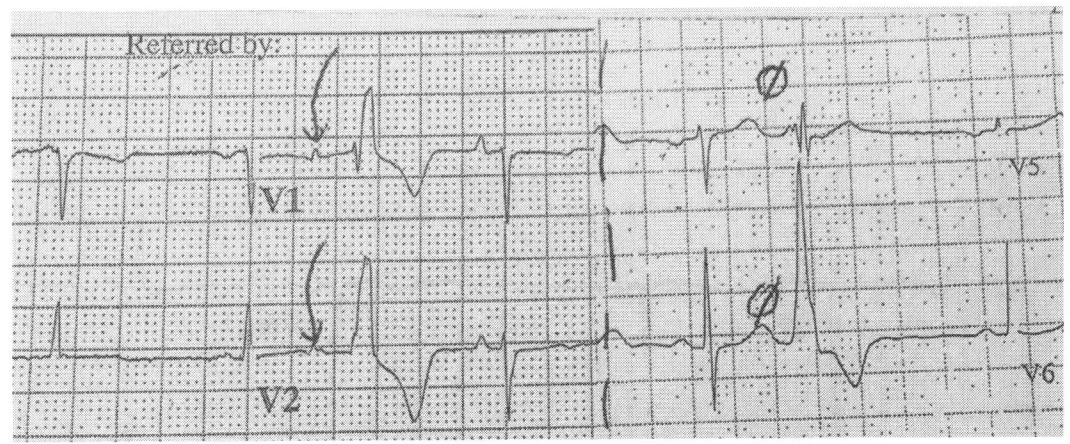

Fig. 34. PAC with aberrancy vs. PVC

The arrows in V1 and V2 point to a small atypical P waves which proves that the subsequent broad QRS complexes are atrial in origin. In the second panel, the broad beat has no antecedent P wave (it would have been seen in the area of the null sign). It is a PVC. When a PVC occurs in the ventricle, the sinus may still fire in the atrium. The normal on-time P wave is often hidden in the large QRS or T of the PVC. It can't cause a normal QRS (the PVC is in the way). The next normal appearing beat, after the PCV, therefore looks late, giving a compensatory pause.

Returning to PAC's, if the premature P wave occurs even earlier, it might land smack on top of the last beat's T wave. Now it finds that neither bundle branch is ready to conduct a new stimulus. With both of them balking, there may be no QRS generated. This is called a nonconducted PAC.

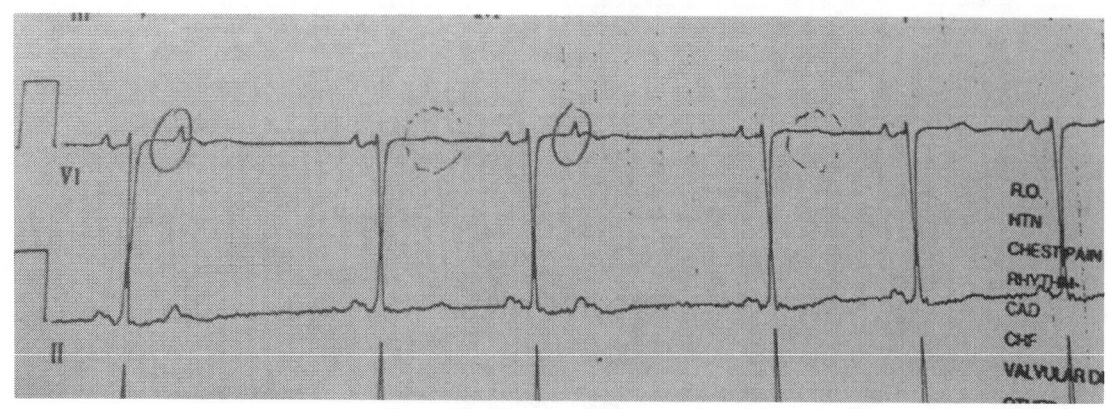

Fig. 35. Nonconducted PAC

In the example above, the first QRS is normal. However, its T wave is distorted by a premature pimple-like P wave which is circled for clarity. It is so early, no QRS ensues due to ongoing ventricular refractoriness in both bundles from the first normal beat. There is a compensatory pause because the premature P can still void the subsequent normally expected sinus impulse. A second and third beat occur normally. Notice the second beat's T wave is not distorted with the pimple-like P wave (dotted circle for emphasis) so a third beat occurs normally. But on the third complex, the premature P is again seen on its T wave, representing another nonconducted PAC, as proven by the subsequent pause. In sinus arrhythmia, seen earlier, there is no ectopic P wave that can be blamed for the pause.

Remember, an ectopic P wave is recognized by a change in axis orientation compared to a normal sinus P. An ectopic QRS is recognized by a broad, abnormal complex, distinct from a bundle branch block in that it arises from the ventricle without a preceding P wave.

On occasion, a "renegade" ectopic atrial or ventricular focus can fire twice in a row. This is called a couplet. If there are three in a row, it is termed a triplet. But if there is sinus rhythm and every other beat is a PAC, or PVC, this is called bigeminy. If a PAC or PVC occurs as every third beat, the condition is called trigeminy.

Sometimes, a single PAC focus can override the sinus node and fire repetitively, controlling the rhythm. Thus, the EKG shows an abnormal P wave before each QRS and is termed "Ectopic Atrial Rhythm" (EAR).

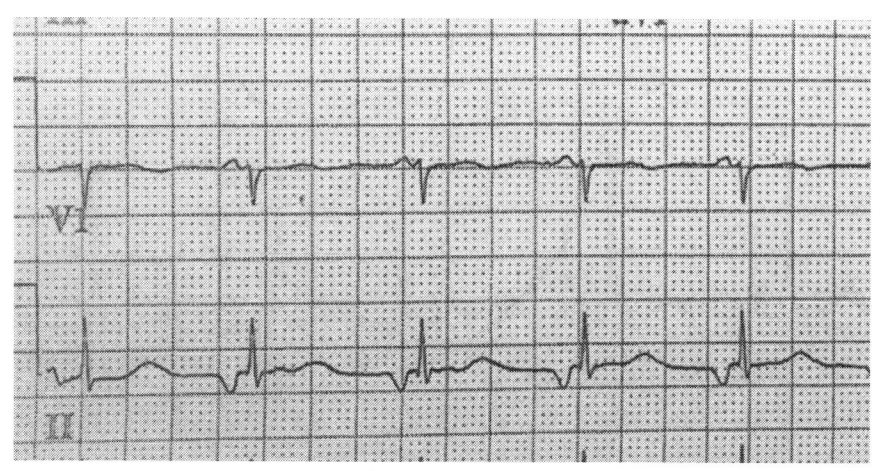

Fig. 36. EAR

This is purely an EKG diagnosis, free of symptoms and undetectable on physical exam. Note the inverted P wave before each QRS in rhythm strip II at the bottom of the trace.

This is, in fact, a favorable situation; if the sinus node relinquishes its role, it is fortunate to have this substitute. Usually, if the sinus node falters, the next backup rhythm is called a junctional rhythm, coming from the Bundle of His, which lies in wait, prepared to fire at 40 to 60 beats per minute. This will be seen later. Unlike the ectopic atrial rhythm above, a junctional rhythm is slower, so as not to compete with the sinus on a day to day basis, and it does not have a preceding atrial contraction. Therefore, EAR has several advantages over a junctional escape: the rate is satisfactory and there is an effective, although ectopic, atrial contraction before the QRS to assure maximal ventricular volume loading due to a preceding "atrial kick".

The next trace shows how a sinus rhythm "morphs" into an EAR.

Fig. 37. NSR becomes EAR

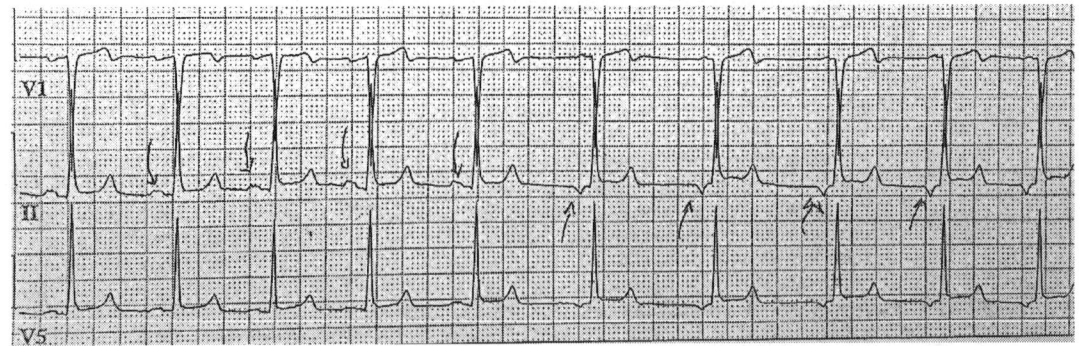

In lead II there is a normal upright sinus P wave for the first few beats (arrows down). Then there is a slight delay between the fifth and sixth QRS, visible to the naked eye. As the sinus node momentarily stalls, the ectopic atrial focus sees a chance to stage a coup and takes over (arrows up).

The following two pictures show analogous situations with respect to a ventricular focus. When a PVC site fires repetitively we see a series of large, aberrant consecutive complexes, the ventricular equivalent of EAR but the QRS complexes are abnormal, not the atrial waves. The rate seen in the example below is 86 beats per minute, not fast enough to fall in the range of tachycardia. Its name is an oxymoron: "Slow Ventricular Tachycardia". A more precise name is "Accelerated Idioventricular Rhythm" (AIVR).

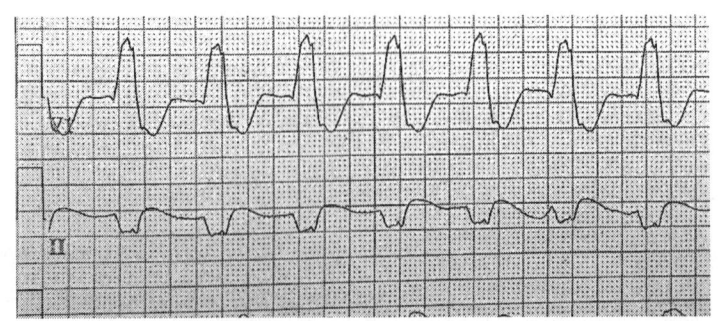

Fig. 38. AIVR

A few words about nomenclature: a sinus rate below 60 bpm is sinus bradycardia, between 60 and 100 bpm is normal sinus rhythm and greater than 100 bpm is sinus tachycardia. When a ventricular rhythm occurs, as above, if below 60 it is called "Idioventricular Rhythm", if between 60 and 100 bpm it is called "Accelerated Idioventricular Rhythm", and if over 100 bpm it is "Ventricular Tachycardia", VT or VTach for short.

We saw a sinus rhythm transform to an EAR two figures ago. Below is a complementary trace showing sinus rhythm morphing into AIVR: Pay attention to rhythm strip II. The first three beats are normal. The last five beats represent AIVR, occurring at a slightly faster rate than the sinus and overtaking it (note how the P waves are "gobbled up", hidden by the broad QRS complexes which fire more quickly). The fourth beat is called a fusion beat, or Dressler beat. It is the love child of a sinus beat heading down the ventricle merging with the broad PVC heading up the ventricle. The fusion beat looks a bit like each "parent".

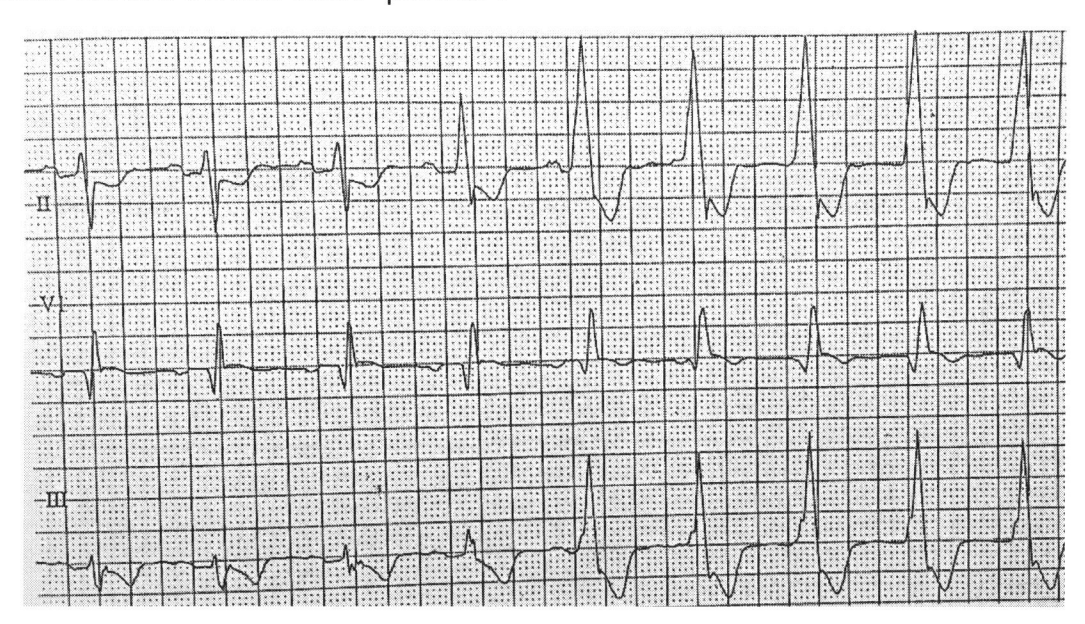

Fig. 39. NSR becomes AIVR

AIVR commonly occurs under one of two conditions. The first is digoxin toxicity in the presence of hypokalemia. Hypokalemia in general is arrhythmogenic. Digoxin, while an electrical suppressant, slowing sinus node firing rate and prolonging AV node conduction, is also an irritant to myocardial tissue, causing inappropriate firing. In the ventricle. This takes the form of AIVR. In the atria, a fast ectopic atrial rhythm can occur at about 160 atrial waves per minute. There is not a 1:1 conduction into the ventricle because of the suppressing effect of the drug on the AV node, so there might be one QRS for every 2 or 3 ectopic atrial waves. This is called "Paroxysmal Atrial Tachycardia with Block" (PAT with block). An example will be seen in Chapter 9.

The second condition which promotes AIVR is the re-establishment of blood flow to an occluded coronary artery; during an acute myocardial infarction muscle is at imminent risk of irreversible ischemic damage. When the artery is opened pharmacologically by a thrombolytic or mechanically by angioplasty, blood flow is immediately restored to the endangered tissue. As if to thank the caregiver for his or her efforts, the tissue gives a "standing ovation"; it fires repetitively as if applauding. AIVR is therefore termed a reperfusion rhythm, often self-limited in duration and, in the midst of reperfusion interventions, is considered a very favorable development.

Continuing an inventory of sites capable of ectopic sources to rhythm, we add the Bundle of His to the list. Belonging to the supraventricular electrical system, it shares properties: it responds to vagal tone, it relies primarily on the right coronary artery's circulation, it gives rise to narrow QRS complexes (unless there happens to be a bundle branch block, delta wave or intraventricular conduction delay downstream).

A junctional rhythm has an intrinsic rate of 40 to 60 bpm, slower than NSR so as not to compete with the latter. It is considered a backup escape rhythm if the sinus stalls. It has a distinct appearance: because this junction lies below the atria and the AV node, when it fires the signal immediately travels down the left and right bundles, giving rise to a QRS. There is no *preceding* P wave. But while the QRS is being generated, the signal also travels backwards, or retrograde, slowly through the AV node. Long after the QRS is recorded, this signal emerges from the AV node into the atria and causes them to contract, from floor to ceiling (the opposite direction of a normal sinus beat). An upside down, retrograde P wave may be seen in the ST segment of the QRS or it might occur with greater delay and be hidden in the T wave. Rarely, if extremely late, the retrograde P may occur after the T wave.

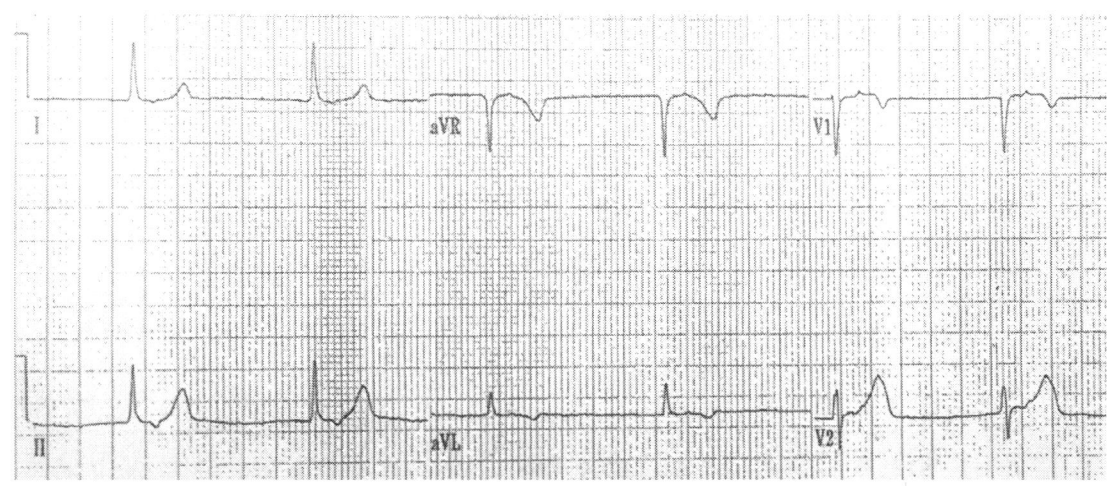

Fig. 40. Junctional rhythm

See fig. 40. The rate is in the 50's. There are no P waves before the QRS. Look carefully at the ST segment in leads II and V1. There are tiny pimple-like retrograde P waves (down in II, up in V1) correlating with the late appearance of atrial activation, delayed by conduction backward up the AV node.

In short, with a junctional rhythm all components of activation occur but instead of P wave followed by AV delay followed by QRS, we see QRS followed by AV delay followed by retrograde P. The atria fire late while the ventricles are already in systolic phase. The higher pressure in the contracting ventricles cannot be overcome by the lower pressure of atrial contraction. As a result, atrial kick does not contribute to filling. In fact, the atrial volume is not strong enough to open the tricuspid and mitral valves and it regurgitates back into the vena cava and pulmonary veins respectively. In the right sided circulation system, this is responsible for cannon A waves on physical exam, a pulsation seen in the jugular vein from regurgitant RA volume.

As stated before, the junction is a backup pacemaker for the sinus node at 40 to 60 bpm. Unfortunately, the sinus node and junction are affected by similar modulating forces. Vagal tone and rate lowering drugs can suppress them both. Therefore, there is yet another backup pacer that lies in wait, less affected by such factors. Not wishing to compete on a daily basis, its backup rate is lower yet, about 21 to 35 beats per minute. This arises from the ventricles (and is therefore wide) and is termed Idioventricular Rhythm, seen below in Fig. 41, slower than *Accelerated* Idioventricular Rhythm (60 to 100 bpm) which we already saw. People may be severely symptomatic by such a low rate and experience syncope or worse.

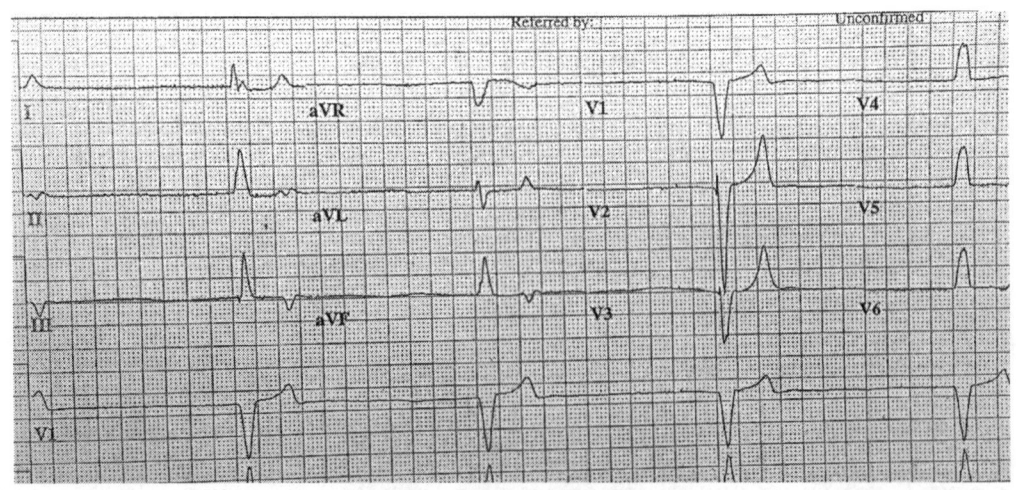

Fig. 41., Idioventricular rhythm (about isoelectric in aVL. Axis near 60)

58

Patients with impaired cardiac function may show signs of further reduced output, presenting with congestive heart failure.

What follows are rhythms revealing increased levels of chaos. As seen, there are many non-sinus pacemakers. If there is one ectopic atrial focus triggered by, say, caffeine, why might there not be 2, 10, 40 or 800 such sites? There can be. If there are a handful of ectopic atrial foci, each firing in its turn, there will be a very irregular rhythm. Each firing site crosses the atria with a different vector and will have its own fingerprint wave direction when viewed by a single lead. This rhythm is called "Wandering Atrial Pacemaker" (WAP) and it is common with lung disease.

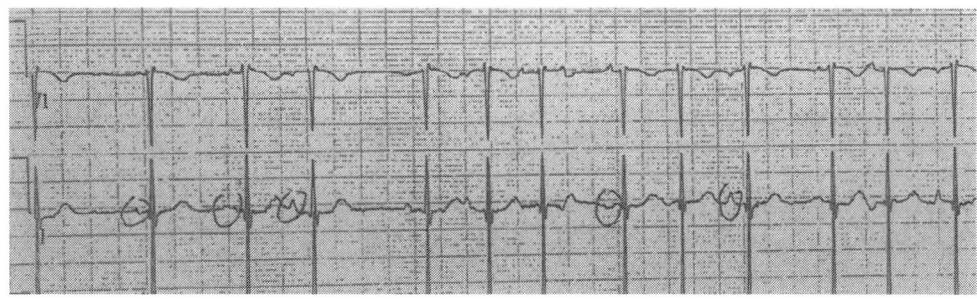

Fig. 42. WAP

In the event of a decompensated pulmonary status, hypoxia and stimulant bronchodilators, WAP may accelerate to rates exceeding 100 beats per minute. We've seen this before: over 100 = new name. WAP becomes Multifocal Atrial Tachycardia (MAT). The distinction is merely one of rate.

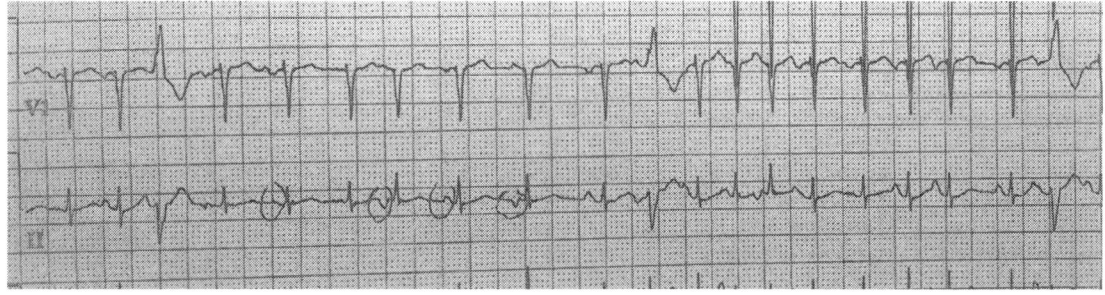

Fig. 43. MAT

These rhythms may mimic atrial fibrillation when taking a pulse due to their fast irregular natures but the EKG will show various ectopic P waves before each QRS (some circled for emphasis). None exist with atrial fibrillation as will be seen shortly. In MAT, note the higher rate. There are even some beats in V1 with a tall rabbit ear, an example of rate-related aberrancy. Some of the morphologically different P waves are circled here as well. When rate is very fast as in the last half of the MAT trace, the large QRS-T complexes may, like skyscrapers, dominate the horizon, making it difficult to see the small, street level P waves. Spreading apart skyscrapers to identify the origins of uncertain rhythms will be seen later when reentrant rhythms are discussed. The same phenomenon of several sites firing randomly can occur with respect to ventricular ectopy. When diverse ones fire, broad beats with variable morphologies will appear in any one given rhythm strip lead. This rhythm is termed "Multifocal PVC's".

Atrial and ventricular fibrillation are the ultimate in ectopy. Imagine a small pond. A youngster has a bucket of stones and repeatedly tosses one at a time into the water. If aimed at the same spot, there will be repetitive, recurring waves of the same morphology. This is sinus rhythm. Next a friend across the pond takes one turn. A single new wave pattern is seen. This is the equivalent of a PAC. More friends join, surrounding the pond, each waiting before taking a turn. Now there are a collection of wave forms as with WAP. Suddenly a rainstorm begins, the children leave and the pond is struck by innumerable drops. The surface quivers and no single tiny wave is able to cross the pond without running into others. There is no unified wave front crossing the pond. This is the model for atrial fibrillation.

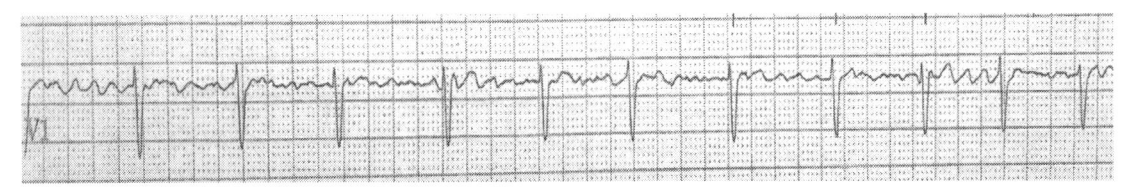

Fig. 44. Atrial fibrillation

The baseline between QRS complexes is constantly covered by "static", mini-attempts to create an effective P wave but unable to do so. This may occur at a rate of 800 to 1000 attempts per minute in the atria. The AV node mediates how many signals cross into the ventricle. Clearly the node cannot allow all to get through. Some impulses never arrive at the node, some arrive but are too weak to cross it, some may cross and the next few try but cannot due to the node's refractory period. The AV node varies in its "mood". Sometimes it is very yielding, as when under sympathetic nervous system drive, allowing many signal to pass, resulting in rapid atrial fibrillation. At other times, it hunkers down, as with increased vagal tone, and is very difficult to cross. Slow atrial fibrillation is the consequence. The AV node can behave like the different judges on a television talent show. Some approve many contestants for the finals and others are less than generous, so scant few go to Hollywood.

Rate control is one problem with atrial fibrillation. If you take a desktop globe of the earth, the depth of atmosphere we can survive in is no thicker than a cellophane wrapping. So it is with heart rate: given the wide range it can take, we are best suited to live in a tiny zone. Atrial fibrillation ventricular response rate is more often like Goldilocks: too fast or too slow rather than just right.

Another problem with atrial fibrillation is loss of atrial kick because there is no organized atrial contraction. Classically the fibrillating atrium is described as a bag of worms. Loss of atrial kick is usually well tolerated unless a patient has significant cardiac dysfunction; such a person may rely heavily on the atrial contribution to maintain adequate cardiac output.

The third major issue with atrial fibrillation is the risk of thromboembolic events. There is a fetal atrial remnant called the left atrial appendage which is a cul-de-sac. Like the GI appendix, it's there to cause trouble (though with all due respect, the GI appendix may act as a reservoir for healthy bacterial flora to reseed the gut, and it has provided generations of surgical residents the chance to hone their skills). Blood can become stagnant in the LA appendage due to lack of organized contraction and clot may form within it. If a bit of clot dislodges from the left atrium, it may embolize anywhere in the systemic circulation, most often in the early branches of the aorta such as the carotids or coronaries. A thrombus the size of a period in this text's font size can produce a neurologically detectable clinical event.

In the ventricle, the analogous rhythm is ventricular fibrillation, triggered by ischemia, fibrosis, inflammation, electrolyte disorders, congenital electrical defects amongst other things. It is fatal if untreated.

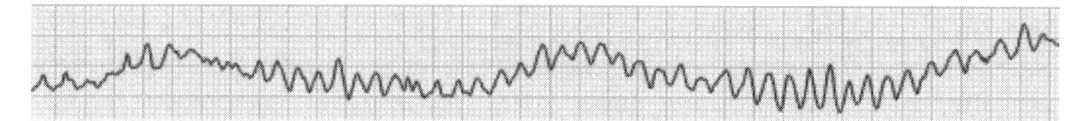

Fig 45. Ventricular fibrillation

Chapter 8: Arrhythmias – Part 2, Reentrant Type

Don't be disappointed: reentry rhythms are few in number. They are generated when an electrical impulse descends through the heart, providing a beat, but at the same time finds itself diverted to loop backwards through some fibers that have different electrical characteristics than neighboring ones. The cycle of anterograde and retrograde is repetitive as well as rapid, each time generating a heart beat.

Following is a simple model to explain why this can happen. Consider the illustration below as a representation of the AV node.

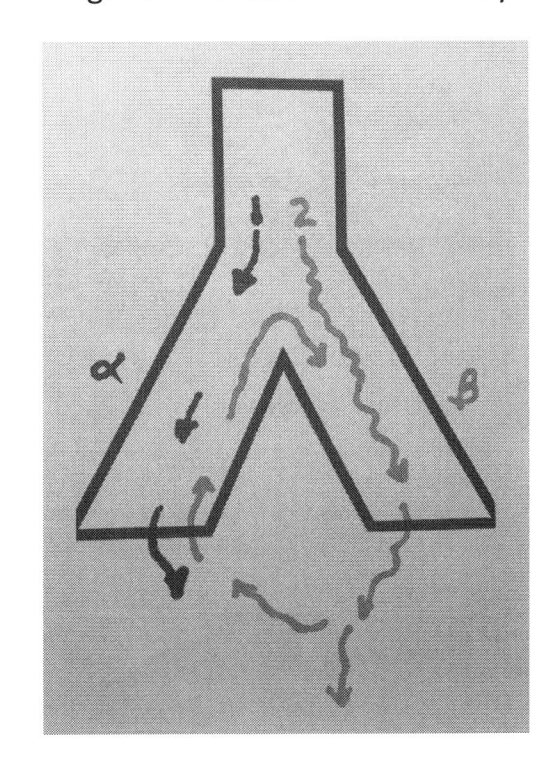

Fig. 46. Mechanism for reentry

There are two paths, alpha and beta, that have different electrical characteristics. Alpha conducts faster than beta but, "working harder" it has a longer refractory period. If a sinus beat enters the top, it preferentially takes the faster alpha path (1) into the ventricle to generate a QRS. It does so repeatedly. But if a sudden premature atrial contraction occurs in the atrium, its signal, arriving early, finds alpha still refractory. It therefore takes slower path 2 down beta. It takes longer to do so. Therefore, by the time it emerges to travel down and create a QRS, alpha has had the extra time to recuperate and "invites" the signal to travel retrograde up it as well. After ascending alpha, the signal finds beta with the shorter refractory period already prepared to accept it for another descent. The cycle is repeated over and over, yielding a rapid and regular recycling, the characteristics of reentrant rhythms.

Beware any two-way street in the heart. It can occur at several levels:

Atrial reentry: When reentry occurs in atrial fibers, there is a cycling round and round the atria at a rate of about 270 to 300 cycles per minute. This back and forth is recorded as repeated up and down waves, the saw tooth tracing we see in atrial flutter. The AV node, due to its intrinsic sluggishness, cannot let every one of these signals through (fortunately) or else the QRS rate would be just as high. At best, every other flutter wave can cross the AV node, yielding a ventricular rate of 135 to 150 beats per minute, a phenomenon called 2:1 flutter. If the AV node is more sluggish than usual due to increased vagal tone or drugs, the ventricular rate will be slower.

AV node reentry: When reentry occurs in the AV node, as illustrated with the diagram, a rhythm called AV node reentry tachycardia (AVNRT) is created. It is also given the less specific name of supraventricular tachycardia (SVT). The name AVNRT is preferred because it is more precise. It will be used hereafter. Depending on the AV nodes tone, which we know is quite variable, the recycling rate can range between 140 and 220 beats per minute.

Ventricular reentry: A third type of reentry occurs in the ventricular tissue, especially when a zone of healthy myocardium lies near a diseased area, such as a zone of ischemia, fibrosis or inflammation. This causes the two regions to behave differently. Reentry in this case creates ventricular tachycardia.

Hail, hail, the gang's all here reentry: The final form of reentry involves everyone - the atria, the AV node and the ventricle- in the case of Wolf-Parkinson-White Syndrome (WPW). As previously discussed, there is an abnormal bypass tract acting as a second AV node. It behaves like the alpha path in the illustration and the normal AV node acts as the beta path. If a current travels from an atrium, down the bypass tract into a ventricle and then up the AV node, a reentry tachycardia is created, wide because each QRS is distorted by a delta wave, mimicking ventricular tachycardia. Because of the bypass tract's longer refractory period, a recycling rhythm may get so fast that the bypass tract is not prepared to accept it, terminating the cycle.

When approaching a rapid regular rhythm, the hallmark of reentry, the first thing to observe is whether the QRS is narrow or broad. If narrow, it is supraventricular in origin.   Fig. 47. Narrow complex tachycardia

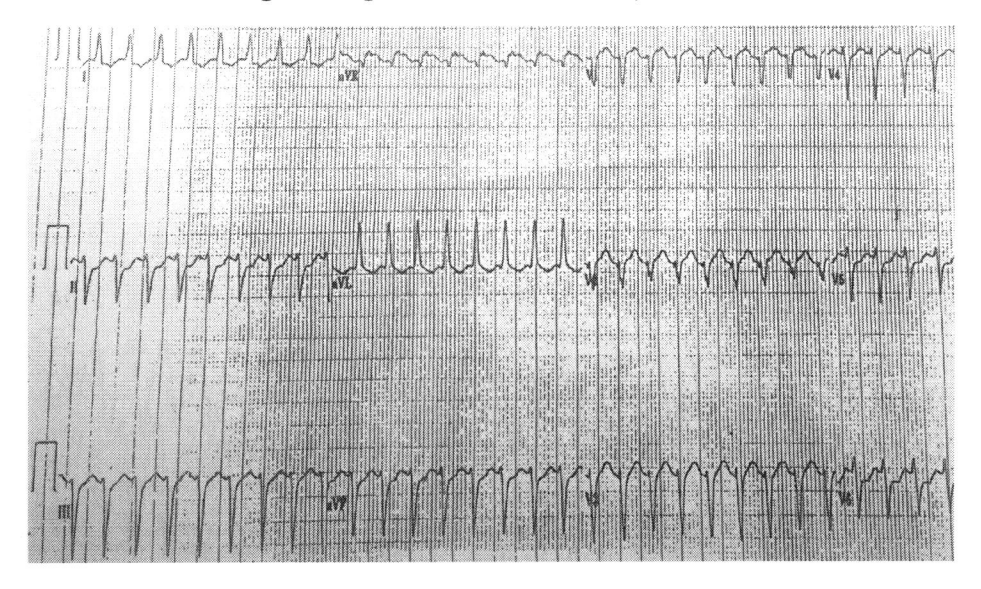

The differential diagnosis is sinus tachycardia, 2:1 atrial flutter or AVNRT. We will see how the QRS rate may help us decide which it is, even when not obvious; sometimes, identifying sinus P waves or atrial flutter waves are not clearly seen because they are small and may be hidden by the rapid and large QRS and T waves which act as skyscrapers dominating the skyline.

If the rhythm is rapid, regular and broad, the differential is ventricular tachycardia or any of the three supraventricular rhythms just discussed if there happens to be a bundle branch block, IVCD or delta wave present that distort the QRS. This is called "supraventricular tachycardia with aberrancy".

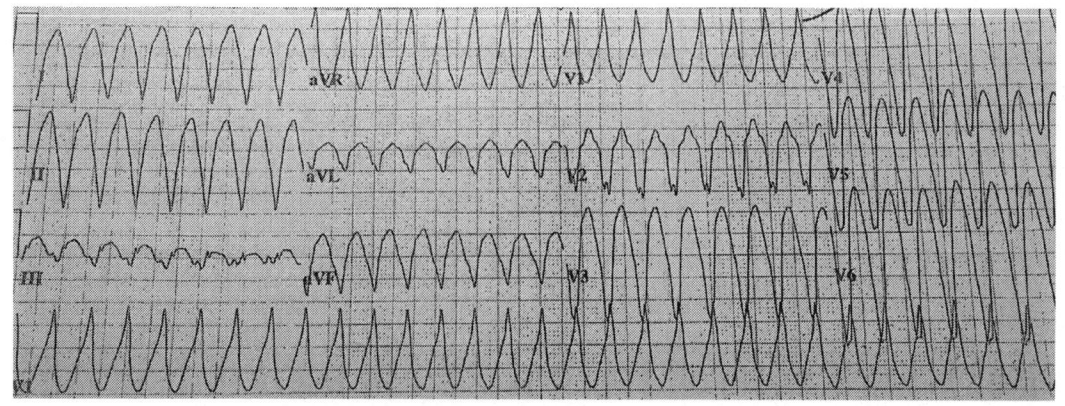

Fig. 48. Broad complex tachycardia

In fig. 47, we find a *narrow* complex, rapid and regular rhythm so it is supraventricular. The patient is an 82-year-old man with chest pain. The rate is 206 bpm. Which rhythm is it? I coin the term "Rule of Rates" to help us. In general, a nontoxic patient can achieve a sinus tachycardia with a maximum of about 225 minus age. This is too high to be sinus in an 82-year old person. Atrial flutter, when highest at 2:1, runs 135 to 150 bpm, again inconsistent with the demonstrated rate. Therefore, it is likely AVNRT.

However, the Rule of Rates is not always reliable, especially in one of two circumstances. The first is if the patient is young. For instance, if this patient is a newborn with hyaline membrane disease, this rate could be consistent with sinus tachycardia at that age. The P waves may be buried by the large QRS and T waves. The second case is when the heart rate is 130 to 160 bpm. These rates can overlap sinus tachycardia, 2:1 flutter and AVNRT in a middle aged adult. In such a case, we can definitively identify the rhythm by seeing what happens when we abruptly slow it (this will be demonstrated later). This I label the "Rule of Deceleration". We will look at some classic examples of the three rhythms under consideration that all present as regular, rapid and narrow.

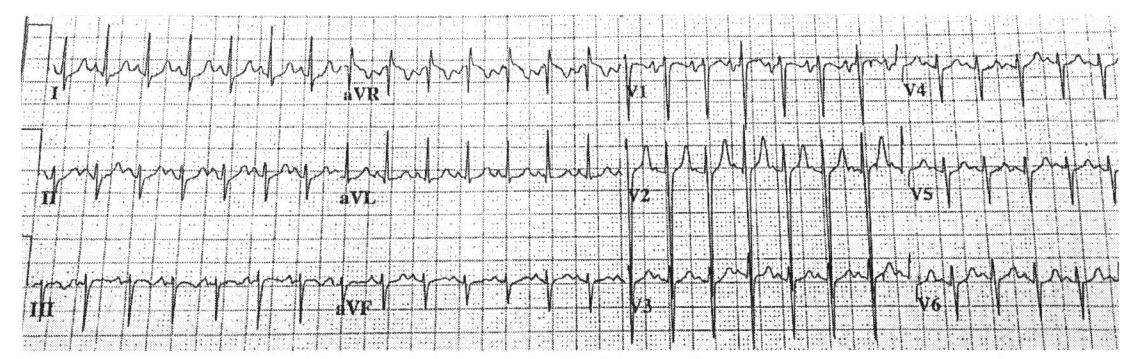

Fig. 49. Sinus tachycardia

In the EKG above, Fig. 49, the patient is a 50-year-old woman with dyspnea. The rate is 170 bpm. This is fast for 2:1 atrial flutter. It is consistent with a sinus tachycardia at this age by Rule of Rates. It might also fall in the wide range of AVNRT, but we clearly see upright P waves in lead II, establishing this as sinus tachycardia. AVNRT originates in the AV node, bypassing the atria, making P waves of this morphology unlikely.

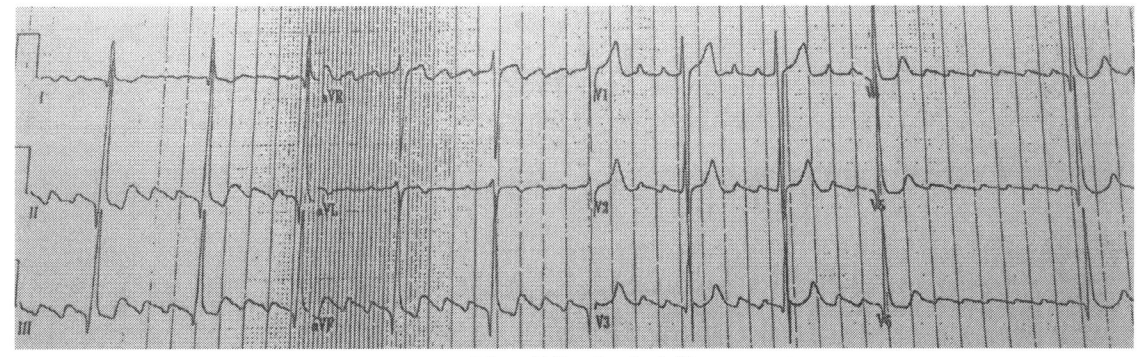

Fig. 50. Atrial flutter

The above trace, Fig. 50, shows a classic rhythm of atrial flutter. In this rhythm the rapid and regular waves are specifically atrial because this is the location of reentry. The EKG shows a typical saw tooth pattern. At a rate approaching 300 bpm, the flutter waves occur about once for every large box on the EKG grid (at standard EKG recording speed of 25 mm/sec, there are 300 large 5x5 mm grids/min). Note the variability of the QRS frequency. This demonstrates how quickly the AV node can block down, yielding fewer complexes at the end of the trace, influenced by variations of sympathetic and vagal tone. Could this be sinus tachycardia with block? No, sinus rate cannot be 300 bpm. Can this be the digoxin toxic rhythm PAT with block? No, the atrial tachycardia in that rhythm, to be seen later, runs about 160 bpm with atrial complexes occurring once every two or three large boxes.

Finally, Fig. 51, below, is a trace in a 68 year old woman with palpitations.

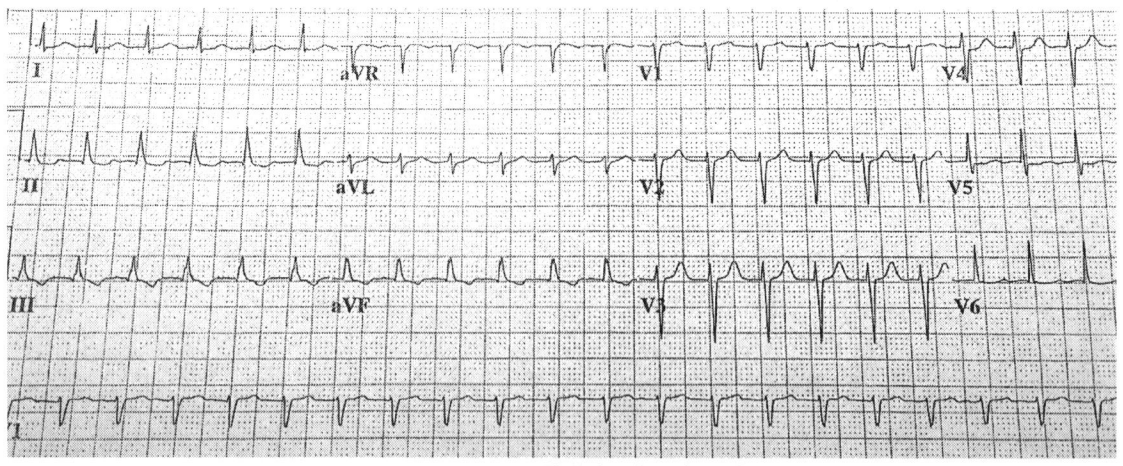

Fig. 51. Which rhythm?

The rate is 141 bpm. The rate is consistent with a sinus tachycardia at her age, 2:1 atrial flutter and a relatively slow AVNRT.

This type of trace is most challenging if one relies on the Rule of Rates. There are no obvious P waves or atrial flutter waves leading to the likely diagnosis of AVNRT but perhaps they are buried. Fortunately, there is another rule, the Rule of Deceleration, that proves definitive in answering the question. This is based on the fact that each of the three rhythms has a different response to a rate lowering maneuver, as will be shown.

Enhancing vagal tone is a physical method and injecting an adenosine bolus is a chemical method that individually can cause this slowdown. Both briefly block the sinus node (rate gets slower) and AV node (harder to cross). These spread out the large QRS-T complexes away from each other, making room to reveal the baseline where atrial mechanisms can be viewed, helping define the original tachycardia.

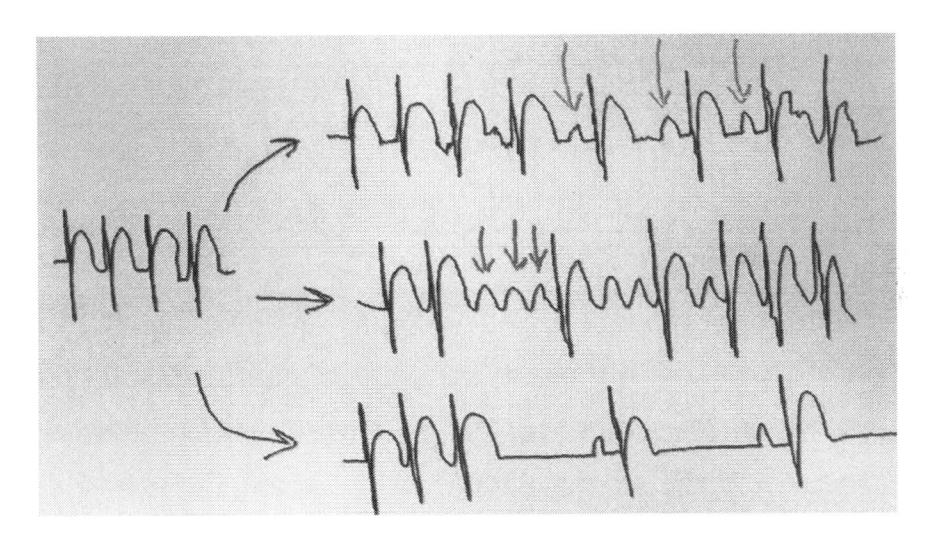

Fig. 52. Three terminations

Refer to Fig. 52. If the tachycardia is sinus in origin (the top case), a vagal surge or an adenosine injection can slow sinus firing rate. The QRS-T complexes "step aside". In the created space P waves will emerge. The downward arrows mark these waves. Again, the effect is brief and shortly thereafter the rate rises again.

In the middle case, if the tachycardia is really 2:1 atrial flutter, the maneuvers blocks the AV node, making it more refractory to the attacking flutter waves. Fewer conduct into the ventricle, decreasing the number of QRS complexes generated. Again, a longer intervening baseline is created revealing the flutter waves in the gap, highlighted by the arrows. Then the rate accelerates again.

In case 3, if the rhythm is AVNRT, a vagal surge or adenosine abruptly blocks the reentry circuit within the AV node, literally jamming the brakes; AVNRT suddenly terminates and usually remains terminated without reaccelerating. Often, there is a pause until the sinus node, having been napping, awakes to resume a sinus mechanism. Remember that the rate lowering maneuver used to block the AV node will also "snuff" the sinus node temporarily, resulting in an initial markedly slow rate that lasts until the influence on the sinus node wears off.

In addition to increasing vagal tone or using adenosine, rate lowering can be effected by medications such as beta blockers, digoxin or the calcium channel blockers verapamil and diltiazem. But oral agents take time to work. Also, they can exert their effects for a long time which is problematic if they slow heart rate too much. These are reasons to initially rely on vagal maneuvers or, if IV access is available, an adenosine bolus.

A vagal surge can be achieved in several ways. Carotid sinus massage (CSM) is performed by rubbing either carotid bulb briefly but vigorously near the angle of the mandible. This should not be performed if there is a carotid bruit or history of cerebrovascular disease because of the theoretical risk of dislodging atherosclerotic plaque. The valsalva maneuver, which also stimulates the vagus nerve, can be attempted by having the patient place a thumb in the mouth, making a tight seal around it and strongly trying to blow without letting air escape. A third way involves the gag reflex: tickle the back of the patient's throat with a soft swab. The alternative, adenosine, can be thought of as a chemical carotid massage. Unlike other pharmaceuticals, it has a half-life of seconds, so an induced bradycardia is very shot lived.

The following are real tracings of termination. Fig. 53 consists of three strips.

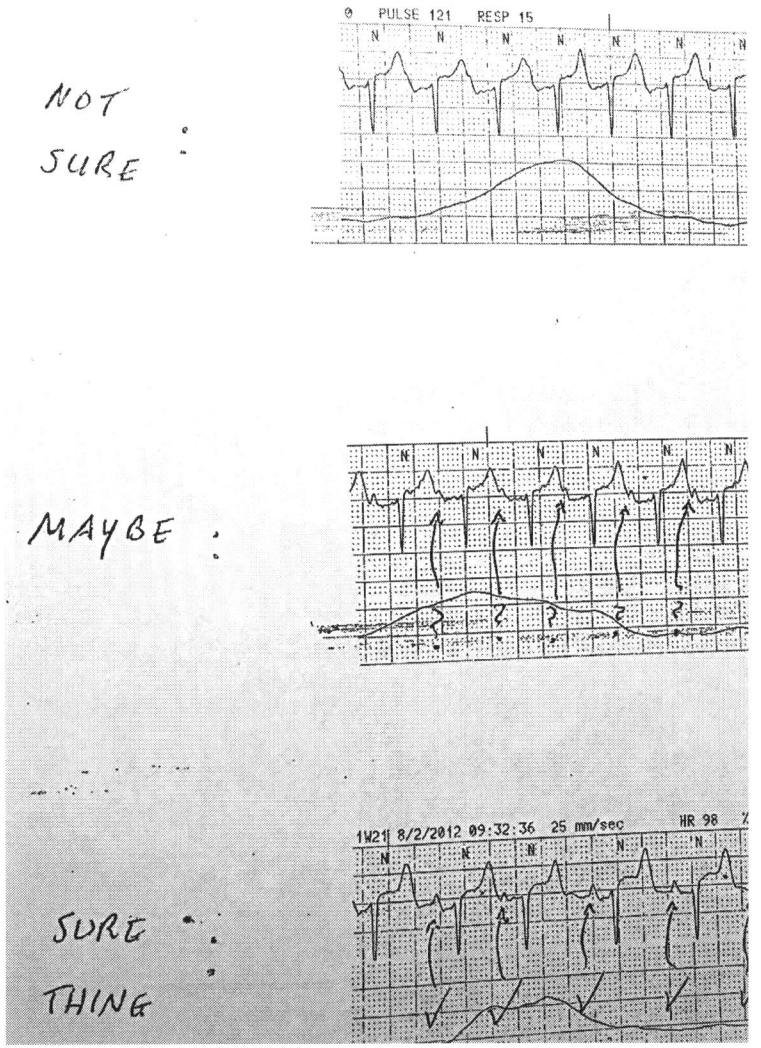

Fig. 53. Slowing reveals sinus mechanism

The first panel shows a narrow complex tachycardia at 121 bpm. Baseline atrial rhythm is not obvious. At first look one might diagnose AVNRT. But when slower in panel 2 there might be P waves poking out on the tail of the previous complex's T wave as indicated by the arrows. When slower yet, the P waves have "room to breath" and declare themselves.

Fig. 54 shows another example of a "Great Pretender".

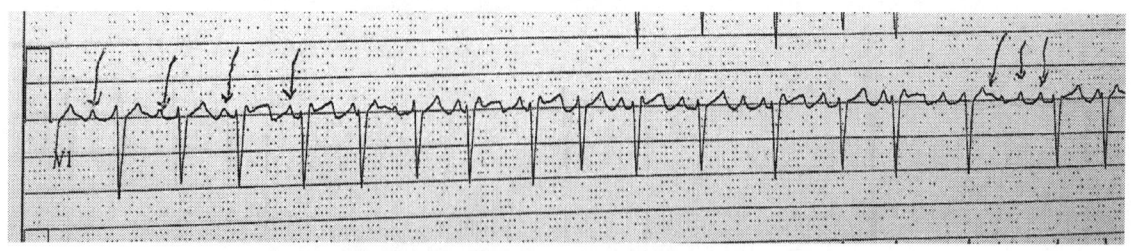

Fig. 54. Slowing reveals atrial flutter

On this rhythm strip there are apparently four P waves and four QRS complexes at the start, suggesting a sinus mechanism. Fortunately, a brief slowing of the QRS frequency at the end of the trace reveals atrial flutter waves at a typical rate of one wave per large box (about 300 cycles per minute). At the start, we are fooled because some flutter waves are buried within QRS and T waves.

A third illustration, fig. 55, is a dramatic, but not unusual, demonstration of abrupt AVNRT termination. AVNRT is a very satisfying rhythm to treat with CSM because when it responds not only has the rhythm been identified by its pattern of termination but it has been successfully treated.

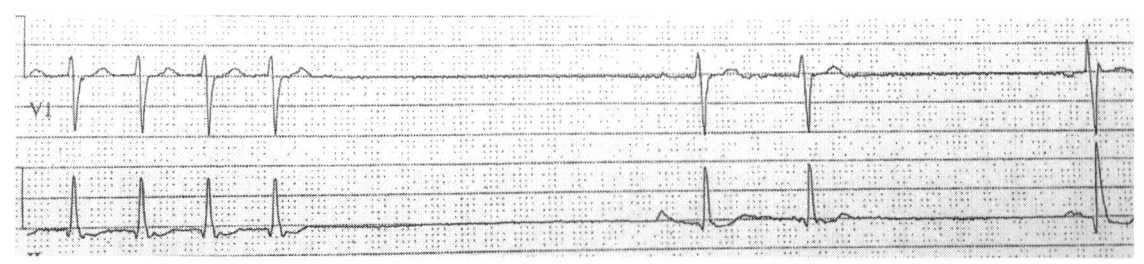

Fig. 55. Slowing reveals an AVNRT origin

Note the stuttering, slow response of the sinus node as it is recruited from rest to assume responsibility for the rhythm. The rate lowering influence that blocked the AV node, breaking the rhythm, also affects the sinus rate which (hopefully) will soon accelerate.

The phenomenon is called Tachy-Brady Syndrome, the dilemma of creating a very slow pulse as a result of efforts to suppress the fast. Some patients with recurrent tachycardia requiring chronic medication suppression might need a backup electronic pacer as a preventative measure against symptomatic asystole if the tachycardia keeps recurring and terminating with such pauses.

I am aware of a patient who was in rapid atrial fibrillation at 180 bpm. He was treated with diltiazem and the antiarrhythmic drug propafenone in an attempt to slow and correct the fibrillation. When the rhythm spontaneously broke it took 30 seconds for the pulse to resume because of the same two drugs' effects on the sinus node. The patient experienced syncope. Fortunately, he was supine in bed at the time and was uninjured. Unfortunately, I was the patient (though I did learn firsthand that asystole is a peaceful way to leave this world). In all seriousness, the risk of asystole, even if self-terminating, goes beyond loss of cerebral circulation and syncope; loss of coronary circulation is also a consequence and with it comes the risk of ischemia-mediated ventricular arrhythmias that could result in sudden cardiac death.

Related to tachy-brady syndrome is Teich's Law of Pulse Rate: "When an arrhythmia is being treated, the average heart rate in the room is 90 bpm."

Specifically, if I walk in on a patient with a bradycardia of 30, my pulse races to 150. If a find the patient in ventricular tachycardia at 160, I go vagal and drop to 20.

Rapid, regular and *broad* tachycardia was previously discussed as either ventricular tachycardia or "supraventricular rhythm with aberrancy", i.e.

when "burdened" with a bundle branch block, conduction delay or delta wave. A very important distinction is that ventricular tachycardia does not respond to vagal stimulating maneuvers. How this assists us is demonstrated on the two following traces. The first reveals a broad regular tachycardia at 135 bpm in a 90-year-old woman.

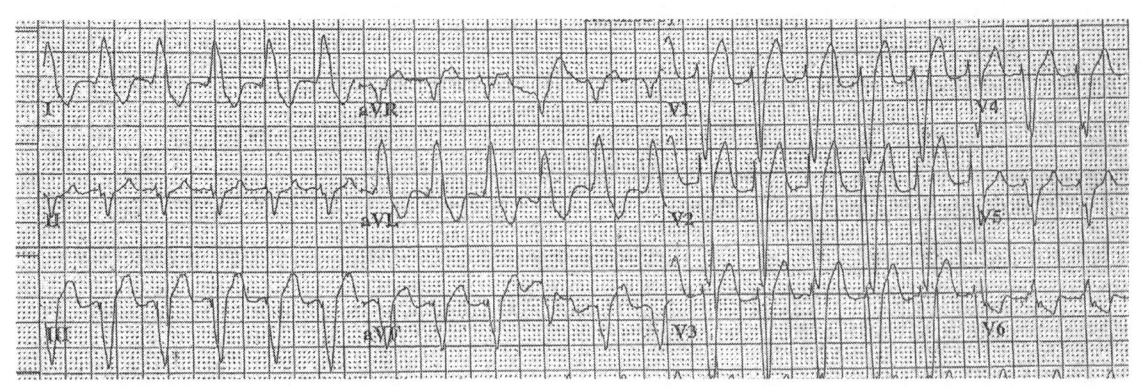

Fig. 56. Broad tachycardia – Supraventricular with aberrancy vs VTach

The diagnosis is uncertain. The wide QRs suggests ventricular tachycardia but this could be a supraventricular rhythm with a left bundle branch block (note the typical deep trough in V1 and reciprocally tall notched complexes in leads 1 and aVL, all characteristic of LBBB). The Rule of Rates is not helpful: 135 bpm is in the realm of possibility for a high sinus tachycardia at this age; 135 bpm could represent 2:1 atrial flutter; it also falls near the lower range AVNRT. Response to a vagal maneuver is seen below and solves the question of origin (ventricular vs. supraventricular), as well as precise mechanism, all at once.

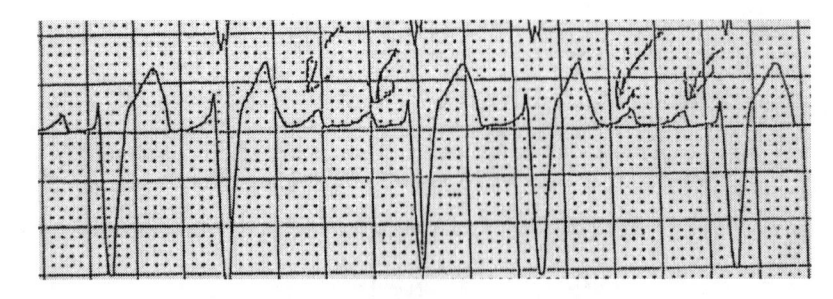

Fig. 57. Slowing reveals atrial flutter with LBBB

Vagal slowing indicates it is supraventricular and not VT. In addition, flutter waves indicated by arrows are seen. Therefore, this is, in fact, atrial flutter with a LBBB.

Chapter 9: Heart Block

Heart block refers to the interruption of normal electrical pathways coursing through the chambers. It can affect several components:

-The sinus node.

-The AV node, called supraventricular, proximal or supra-His block.

-The three ventricular fascicles (the right bundle and the two fascicles of the left bundle), called distal or infra-His block.

Unexpected sinus pauses or cessation (called sinus arrest) can be seen as a result of rate lowering drugs, ischemia, elevated vagal tone, hypothyroidism and age-related decline in function. If the sinus node halts long enough, a junctional rhythm is the first expected backup, arising from the Bundle of His at a rate of 40 to 60 bpm with a narrow QRS. An example was seen earlier in Fig. 40.

AV nodal block can occur for the same reasons as sinus. Lyme's disease can also cause AV block. It's seen in three progressive degrees: first, second and third. The last is also called complete AV block. There is good news and bad news. The good news is that the worst case scenario, complete shutdown of the AV node, will hopefully result in a decent junctional escape rate at 40 to 60 bpm, compatible with survival. Because the AV node resides above the Bundle of His, AV block is also called *supra*-His block. The bad news is that the AV node, as a single focus, can go to complete shutdown in a matter of seconds or minutes depending on the cause.

In comparison to this, distal heart block also has good news and bad news. The good news is that one is dealing with three individual fascicles, not a single site as in the case of the AV node. It usually takes many months to years for all three fascicles to fail sequentially. The bad news is that this block happens downstream from the Bundle of His. It's called *infra*-His block so a junctional escape isn't useful; it has no paths available to the ventricle. In this situation, a distal slow idioventricular rhythm is the escape mechanism and, at 21 to 35 bpm, may cause significant symptoms or death.

The three degrees of AV block are a function of progressive fatigue. As an analogy consider a session at a gym performing bicep curls. The P wave is the trainer's command; the PR interval represents the timing of my response. Using very light weight, each time I am asked to perform a set, I do so promptly. This is the equivalent of normal sinus rhythm with a normal PR interval of 3 to 5 mm boxes, 120 to 200 msec.

Next, an additional challenging amount of weights is added. With each command, I perform a set but it takes me longer to finish it than it did before. This represents first degree AV block, a PR interval longer than before, exceeding 200 msec, but consistently the same with each beat.

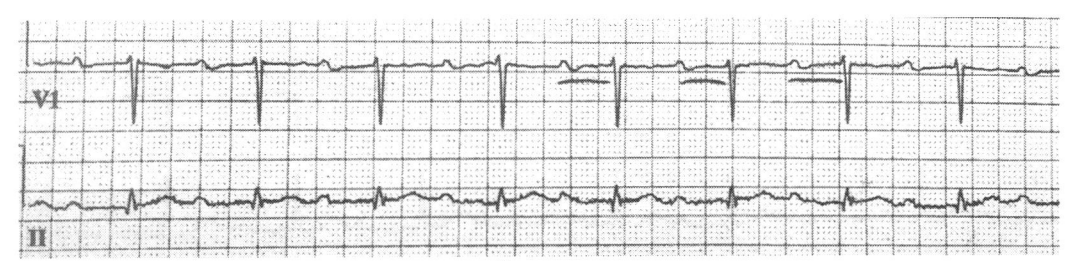

Fig. 58. 1ˢᵗ degree AV block

In the strip above, the PR interval is underlined and uniformly the same but longer at about 400 msec (two large boxes).

With even greater weight, it takes me longer and longer to perform in response to each command until I fail to respond and take a breather. Patiently, my trainer allows this but then resumes the session. However, I continue the same pattern, lengthening my response with each set until down the line I take another pause. This is second degree AV block: longer and longer responses with periodic pauses. It is also termed Mobitz Type 1 block or Wenckebach Block.

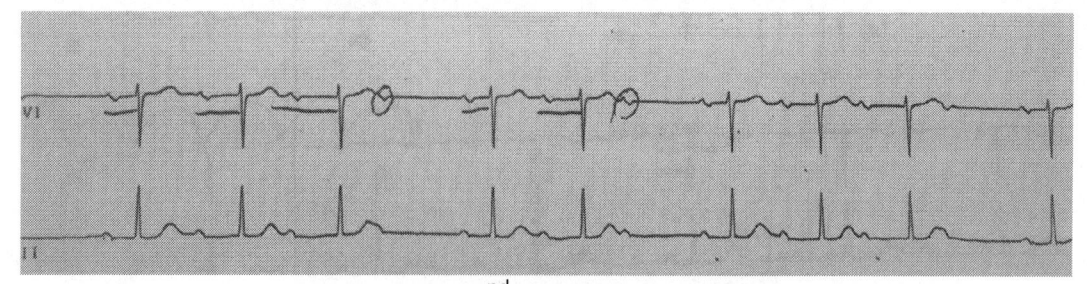

Fig. 59. 2nd degree AV block

In the above sample, note the progressive delay as indicated by the lengthening underscored line until a P wave (circled) goes unheeded. The mantra is "long, longer, longer, blocked" and then the cycle begins again. The blocked P wave need not always occur after the same number of successfully conducted cycles. In the first set there are 4 P waves and 3 QRS complexes ("4 to 3 Wenckebach). In the second set we see "3 to 2 Wenckebach". It is important to note that the *P waves are always on time* in AV block of all degrees; the delay is in the AV node. This is in distinction to a vasovagal reaction where AV delay gets longer and longer and P waves get further and further apart as well. Remember to look for P wave regularity when you see an arrhythmia like this because Wenckebach is pathologic but a vagal reaction is not (as when a patient on telemetry bears down for a bowel movement or gags briefly).

Finally, the weight is so challenging that I dismiss my trainer. The instructions come at a regular interval but I do my sets on my own, slower frequency, deaf to the commands. This is third degree or complete AV block. With complete AV node block there is dissociation of P waves from QRS complexes. P waves fire according to the depolarization rate of the sinus node. The impulses can't pass through the AV node. The downstream

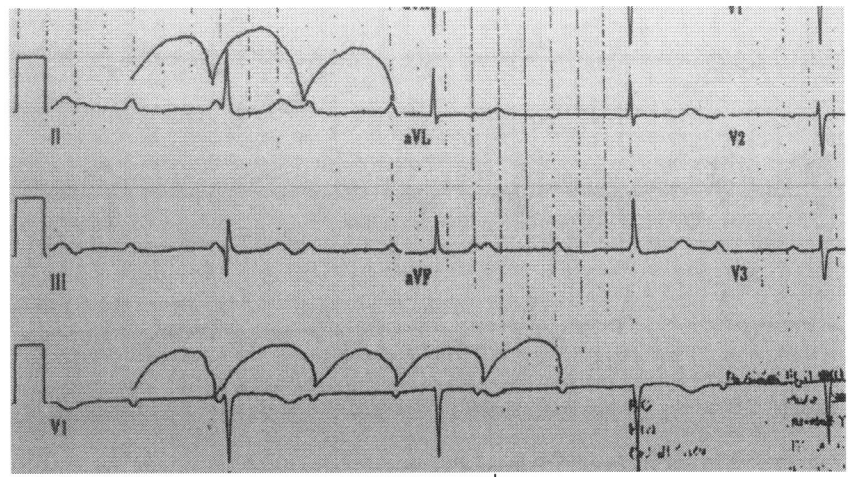

Fig. 60 Complete 3rd degree AV block

Bundle of His fires at its intrinsic rate of 40 to 60 bpm, oblivious to the actions of the sinus because the AV node is now a brick wall in-between. The above trace shows P waves, indicated by the cascading markings, with the QRS "marching to the tune of a different drummer".

While discussing AV block, the time is appropriate to introduce the following trace which is an example of an iatrogenic disorder

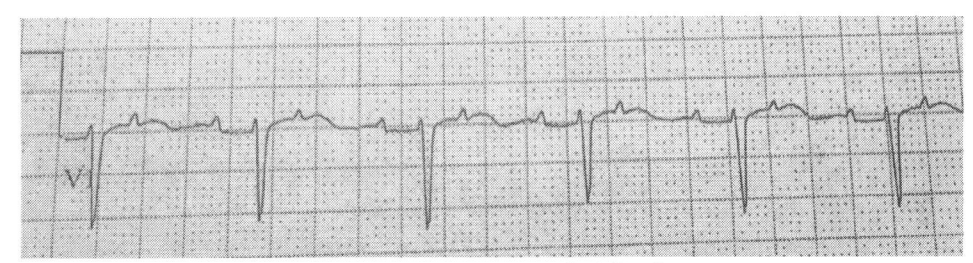

Fig. 61. PAT with block

In this trace taken from an 85-year-old patient there are <u>atrial</u> events at about 160 bpm.

These are fast for sinus origin at this age, the maximum estimate being 140 bpm, yet too slow for atrial flutter which occurs at about 300 waves per minute. This in fact is a trace resulting from digoxin toxicity in the presence of hypokalemia. Recall digoxin irritates myocardial tissue, triggering it to fire ectopically and inappropriately. In the ventricle the equivalent rhythm is AIVR (accelerated idioventricular rhythm, as seen before). In the atrium the rhythm is called paroxysmal atrial tachycardia (PAT). The digoxin also slows conduction in the AV node so not every atrial wave gets through. The name of the rhythm becomes "PAT with block".

An introduction to distal heart block has been presented earlier in this chapter and in the chapter on the QRS complex. Briefly, for review, this occurs slowly over months to years as the three distal fascicles (right bundle branch, left anterior and left posterior fascicles) falter one by one, usually from age, fibrosis or ventricular ischemic injury. Only one fascicle is needed to bring a current from the atria to the ventricles.

Imagine a person with a cane (just used for show). The legs and cane represent the three electrical branches. If the cane is removed (RBB or either fascicle) the person remains standing. This is "unifascicular block". If, in addition, one leg is disabled, this is the equivalent of "bifascicular block" (RBBB with LAHB – or RBBB with LPHB – or LBBB alone). In this instance the remaining leg is of paramount importance for if it fails P waves cannot reach the distal ventricles due to trifascicular block and the slow dangerous idioventricular rhythm will result. Notice that each of the three definitions of bifascicular block contains one type of bundle branch block or the other.

A patient with bifascicular block should always have some form of prolonged monitoring (several methods are available on an outpatient setting) and be asked to report any symptoms such as unexplained dizziness or syncope because these events might reflect transient trifascicular block. There are even invasive electro physiologic studies to study the health of the three fascicles. If the third fascicle fails even once, missing a single QRS, the rhythm is called Mobitz Type II. In such an instance, consideration to an artificial pacemaker should be given before the transient loss of function becomes permanent. Here is an example.

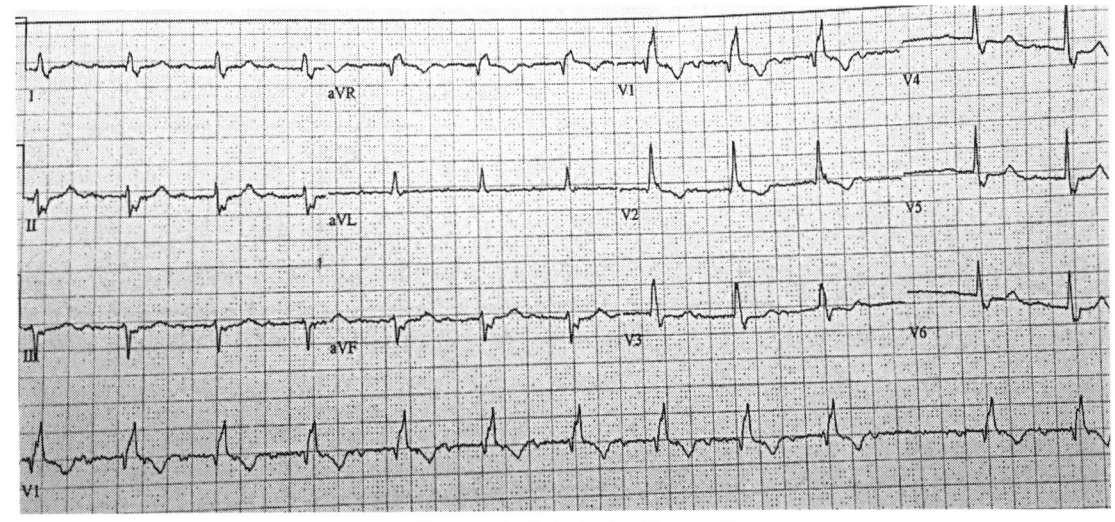

Fig. 62. Mobitz Type II

Remember that bifascicular block is a prerequisite for Mobitz II and all forms of bifascicular block contain a bundle branch block. Therefore Mobitz II must contain a wide QRS. If a narrow QRS is present, the block cannot be distal. Note the baseline sinus rhythm with long PR. The rabbit ears in V1 indicate a RBBB. The left axis (negative in lead II, net positive in lead I) indicate a left anterior hemi block. Together the two represent bifascicular block. At the end of V1,2 and 3 near the switch to V4,5 and 6, there is an "orphaned" P wave best seen on the V1 rhythm strip running across the bottom – no QRS is generated. This is a one-time failure of the last branch. If permanent, the slow idioventricular (IVR) rhythm will develop (Fig. 63).

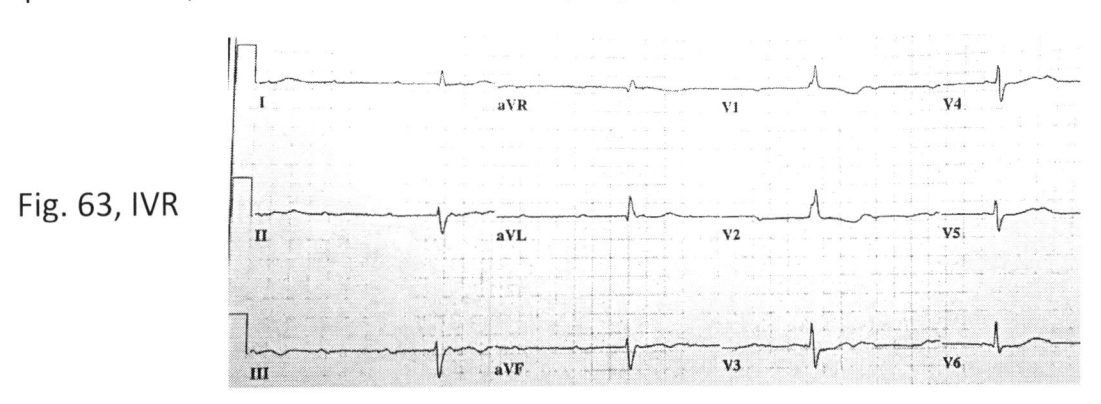

Fig. 63, IVR

Chapter 10: Ischemic Patterns

Ischemia is a state where an organ receives insufficient blood supply and metabolism is compromised primarily due to the lack of oxygen and glucose. Within minutes, cellular death occurs, a condition called necrosis. While the heart is the source of circulation, its muscle mass (particularly that of the left ventricle) is so thick that the blood within the four chambers is not enough to feed the walls through and through. Therefore, the coronary arteries which cover the heart's surface send branches deep into the muscular layer to meet metabolic demands. Insufficient flow most often occurs from atherosclerotic obstruction of these arteries. Other causes can be shock with poor perfusion pressure and spasm of the blood vessels. Damage can also occur from acidosis, infections and trauma. This chapter deals with atherosclerosis.

When the coronary artery endothelial lining is injured as with hypertensive shearing forces, long term results of diabetes and smoking and hyperlipidemia, the mediators of inflammation and scar formation are recruited. Infiltration by lipids attracts macrophages to engulf the fatty material, forming foam cells which trigger a series of events responsible for the formation of plaque which is a complex lesion involving cholesterol, cell proliferation, collagen, fibrosis, new vessels and calcium. These lesions can be focal and, like a hose pinched at a point, can reduce available blood supply downstream. A person may have significant narrowing of an arterial lumen, up to about 75%, and remain asymptomatic; but at some point the lumen's compromise, like a tightening noose, is enough to cause the symptom of angina, usually when the heart is called upon to work harder as with exercise. The increased heart rate, blood pressure and wall tension accompanying this type of activity leads to a greater demand for coronary blood flow. Without adequate supply, lactic acid can be produced and, unless treated, ischemia results in permanent damage. Goals are to 1) control and eliminate risk factors if possible, 2) reduce cardiac demand with medication that lower heart rate, blood pressure and wall tension, 3) increase blood flow by trying to relax the muscle in the walls of the coronary arteries pharmacologically, 4) pool blood in the veins with nitrates to reduce returning volume thereby reducing wall stress in the heart and 5) reduce plaque mechanically by angioplasty and stenting if medical therapy is inadequate. If these fail, consider bypass surgery especially if multiple coronary arteries are involved.

The bulk of coronary circulation is devoted to the left ventricle because of its mass and workload so this chamber is particularly susceptible to ischemia. One can understand the dynamics of ischemia by considering the LV as a hollowed out pumpkin, the cavity being the LV chamber space. The coronary arteries cover the surface of the pumpkin and send branches into the deep rind. If a plaque limits coronary blood flow to a significant degree temporarily because of a new demand such as exercise, there is not enough circulation downstream from the blockage to percolate into the deepest levels of myocardium. In the heart this layer is called the subendocardial zone (because it abuts the inner lining of the LV cavity) and is most susceptible to "subendocardial ischemia" also called "non-transmural ischemia".

Because some patients don't feel classic angina even when ischemia is present, and because not all chest pain is due to coronary insufficiency, the EKG is a helpful diagnostic tool to help assess whether or not a cardiac circulatory problem exists.

When a zone of myocardium is ischemic, it may still participate in systolic contraction but during diastolic relaxation, as healthy tissue returns to electrical baseline, the ischemic zone lags. This difference in electrical status creates a diastolic "current of injury", directed towards the afflicted area. To the EKG leads overlying this ischemic territory, the current is heading away from them towards that inner layer of the pumpkin. This creates ST depression because the ST segment correlates with early diastole.

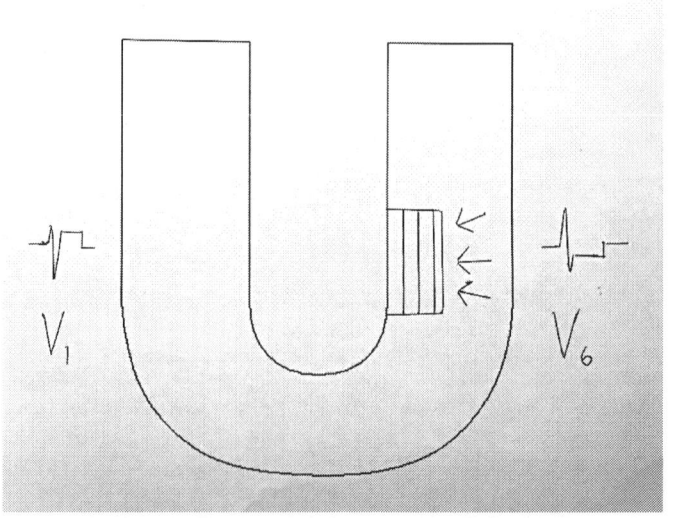

Fig. 64. Subendocardial ischemia

In the diagram, the LV cavity is represented by the letter U. To the reader's right is the patient's left lateral wall, to the left is the septum. The deep, subendocardial wall is ischemic (striped zone). The current of injury directed toward it is indicated by the arrows, heading away from an overlying lead, V6 in this case. Note the ST depression in V6. On the opposite side of the heart, one might see the current of injury directed toward *that* area's overlying lead (V1 in this instance) leading to reciprocal ST elevation there, but this is often subdued due to the distance from the ischemic zone.

Most of the time ST depression is reversible. With rest, as myocardial demand for blood subsides, circulation through a partially occluded vessel percolates through the residual lumen opening and this may be enough to meet metabolic requirements downstream once more.

ST depression by itself is not specific for subendocardial ischemia. Non-ischemic conditions may be responsible for it such as left ventricular hypertrophy, left bundle branch block, digoxin, hyperventilation or electrolyte abnormalities. One must always correlate the clinical status of the patient when interpreting an EKG. With the right story, setting or physical findings, suspicion is heightened that the finding is a true positive. In addition, there are criteria for the degree of ST depression that also raise concern. The point where the QRS ends and the ST line begins is called the "J Point" (J for junction). It should be at least 1 mm depressed from baseline (defined as the horizontal level between beats) and remain at least 1 mm depressed for a minimum of 80 msec (2 mm across).

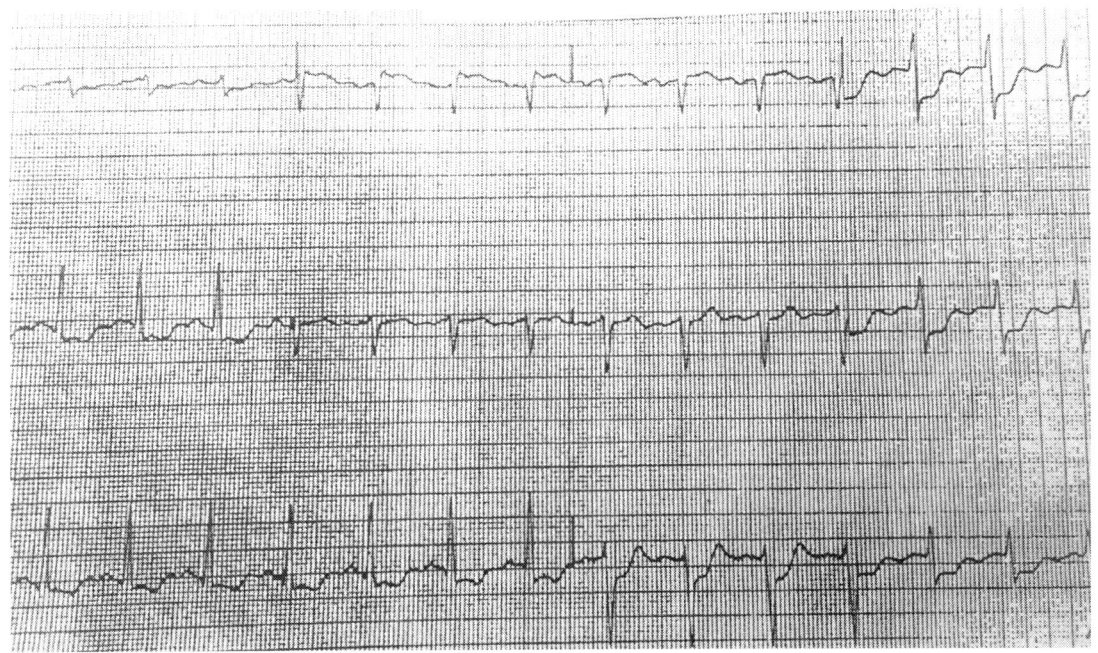

Fig. 65. ST depression

In the tracing seen in Fig. 66 there is widespread ST depression. As an example, examine V5 (last column, middle row). Note where the QRS ends and the ST segment begins. This is the J point and it is about 5 mm lower than baseline. Because it is horizontal, 2 mm later it remains similarly depressed, meeting the above criteria.

Possible variations can include the following: 1) the J point is several millimeters depressed but rises steeply so that 80 msec later it is back to baseline. This is called "J point depression with rapidly upsloping ST segments" and is a common, normal pattern seen in young people with exercise induced tachycardia; 2) the J point and the follow-up point are depressed but one or both do not exceed 1 mm. This is called non-specific ST depression. This can be seen in lead V2 in Fig. 66 (third column, middle row). Is it important? It depends on the status of the patient's symptoms, history and the presence or absence of such changes on prior routine EKGs.

Returning the a partially obstructive atherosclerotic plaque, events can deteriorate rapidly if the surface is disrupted. A protective fibrous cap overlying the lesion may ulcerate, hemorrhage may occur within it or the edge may lift off as happens on the border of a scab. Exposure of collagen within the core of plaque to circulating blood causes platelets to engage in "The Dance of the Four A's": they are **A**ttracted to the site, sensing an injury; they **A**dhere to the local endothelium; they are **A**ctivated resulting in release of granule contents containing mediators of inflammation; and they **A**ggregate, binding to each other by glycoproteins to form a platelet plug. Breakdown of platelet membranes result in activation of the arachidonic acid pathways, creating prostaglandins, prostacyclin, thromboxane and leukotrienes that modify and regulate the response. The coagulation cascade is triggered resulting in fibrin clot which, with the platelet plug, can completely occlude the artery. This is a medical emergency because, if left untreated, the full thickness of heart muscle downstream is in jeopardy of rapid and irreversible suffocation and destruction in a matter of a few hours. This is called "transmural ischemia" and the consequence can be a transmural myocardial infarction. Aggressive inpatient therapy is needed, such as urgent angioplasty or thrombolytic therapy.

Fortunately, the EKG changes its appearance to alert the clinician of this emergency by displaying a different hallmark, ST segment elevation (at least 1 mm). The explanation for the change in pattern is shown in Fig. 66.

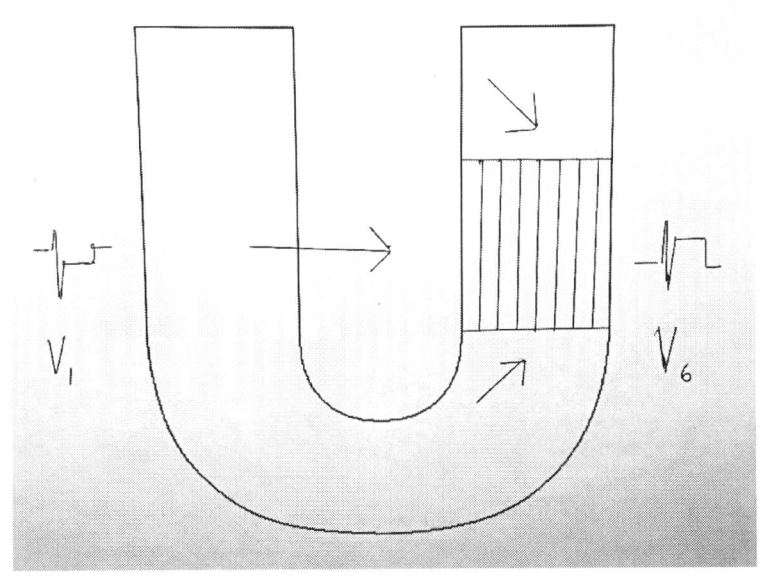

Fig. 66. Transmural ischemia

In the drawing, the lateral LV wall zone of transmural ischemia is indicated by the striped segment. Recalling that the current of injury is aimed at the compromised tissue, it is now directed *towards* the overlying lead (V6) from the surrounding non-affected tissue, reversing direction compared to subendocardial ischemic conditions. As such the ST segment is elevated in

V6 and its neighbors with reciprocal ST depression on the opposite side of the heart (V1) which sees the current retreating.

Just as ST depression need not always represent subendocardial ischemia, ST elevation may be an indicator of conditions other than an imminent myocardial infarction, leading to different, and sometimes no, intervention. ST elevation variations can be classified as being "the good, the bad and the ugly".

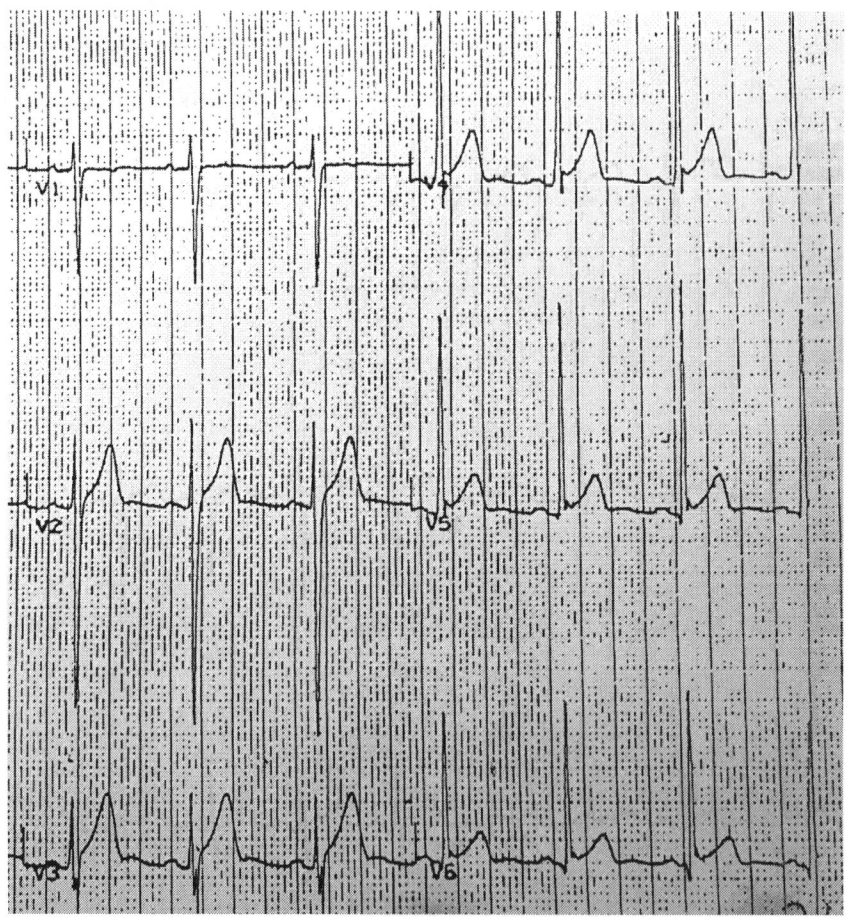

Fig. 67. Early repolarization

Fig. 67 demonstrates the "good" ST elevation. The patient is a 17-year-old asymptomatic young man obtaining an EKG as a routine preoperative study. Only the precordial leads are shown. Note the ST elevation in these leads as well as the generous voltage. The latter is not unexpected in a young thin male with little subcutaneous fat within the chest. The ST elevation is called early repolarization and, in this clinical setting, is of no concern. As the name suggests, the T wave is already on the upslope before there is a flat ST segment and it is a variant of normal in the young. A very characteristic finding is the scooping morphology of the wave as it transitions from QRS to T wave, similar to the swoosh logo of a well known sports apparel company. Look at V4, V5 and V6.

Be careful not to assume the innocence of this pattern. While not unexpected in asymptomatic youth, the swoosh in an older patient with typical ongoing anginal chest pain should be considered a marker of transmural ischemia until proven otherwise.

The "bad" form of ST elevation is shown in Fig. 68, the variant seen in pericarditis. ST elevation is best seen in lead II, V4, V5 and V6.

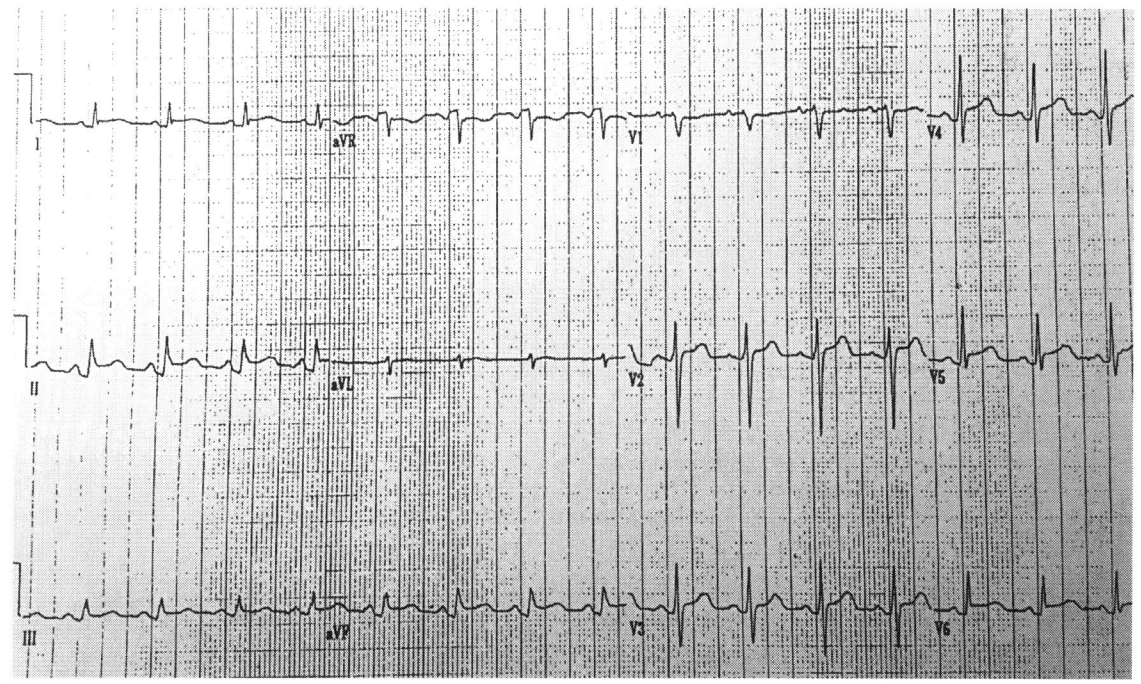

Fig. 68. Pericarditis

The patient is a 65-year old man with lung cancer who presented with sharp, positional chest discomfort radiating to the left shoulder region. His EKG is typical of pericarditis, in this case due to tumor erosion into the pericardial sac, allowing blood to accumulate in the space. A bloody pericardial effusion, even if tiny, can trigger a sterile inflammatory response which is the cause of his disorder.

The pericardial sac covers the lower chambers of the heart and extends up to cover part of the atria. While not ischemic in origin, with pericarditis there is inflammation over the entire surface of the heart. The current of injury is directed from myocardium to surface globally, accounting for widespread ST elevation in anterior, lateral and inferior leads. As the pericardium reflects up and over the atria, from bottom to top, the current of injury over these chambers is directed toward the spine, away from the surface of the chest. The atria have T waves too small to be seen on a standard EKG but their ST segment is incorporated in the PR segment. Heading *posteriorly*, the atrial current of injury appears as ST depression following the P wave when viewed by the normally *anteriorly* placed EKG lead wires. PR depression is a good indicator of pericarditis and is best seen in leads II and aVF on our trace.

Remember that a good history and physical exam will also help establish the diagnosis by the quality of pain and presence of a pericardial friction rub respectively. If in doubt, immediately check cardiac enzymes, seek out an older EKG for comparison and consider an echocardiogram which may support a diagnosis of pericarditis by the finding of a pericardial effusion or a diagnosis of myocardial infarction by a regional wall motion abnormality. Empiric thrombolytic therapy is ill-advised without a sure diagnosis; if pericarditis is the true event, a thrombolytic agent could cause hemorrhage into the pericardial space, prompting life threatening cardiac tamponade.

The "ugly" form of ST elevation is that which represents a true myocardial infarction. Usually a specific lead cluster – anterior, inferior or lateral- will be involved but sometimes, in the case of multivessel coronary disease, where an abrupt occlusion closes one vessel and its collateral vessels to other occluded arteries, the changes can be widespread. This can also occur with a left main coronary artery occlusion. Examples follow.

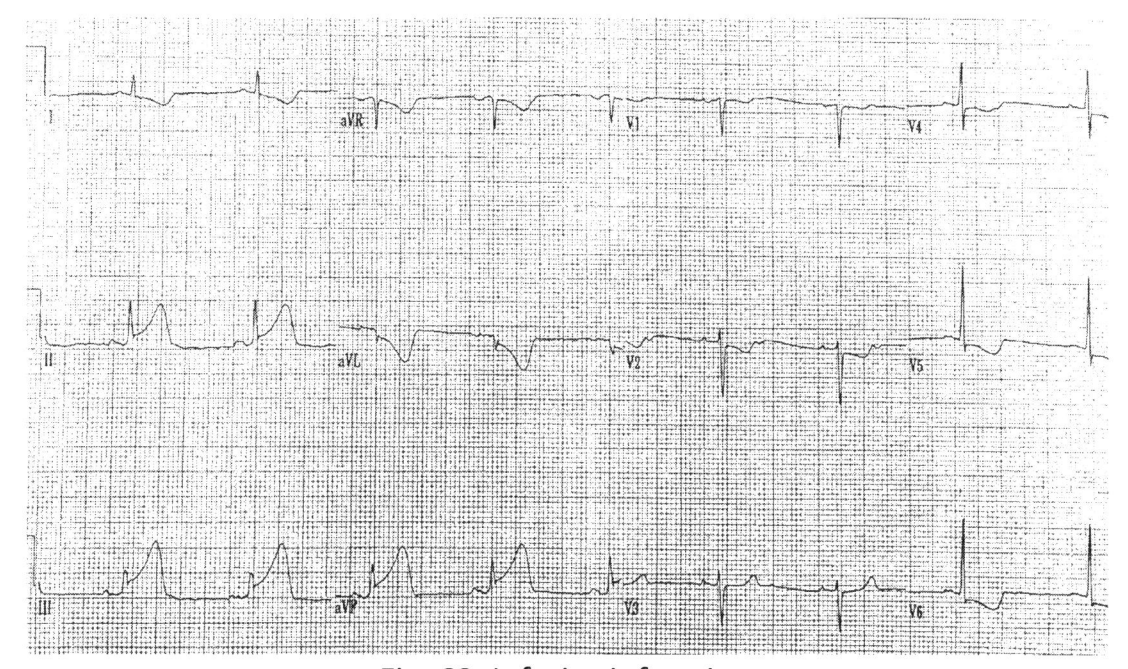

Fig. 69. Inferior infarction

In Fig. 69 inferior ST elevation is seen in leads II, III and aVF indicating an inferior wall myocardial infarction, usually as a result of right coronary artery occlusion. Note the reciprocal ST depression seen by leads that record walls located away from the active ischemia.

This second of the two traces shows massive myocardial damage with permanent features at an advanced stage. The ST segments cove up and over, a pattern called "tombstoning"; this is seen particularly well in the lateral precordial leads, V4, V5 and V6. The Q waves in the V leads are also

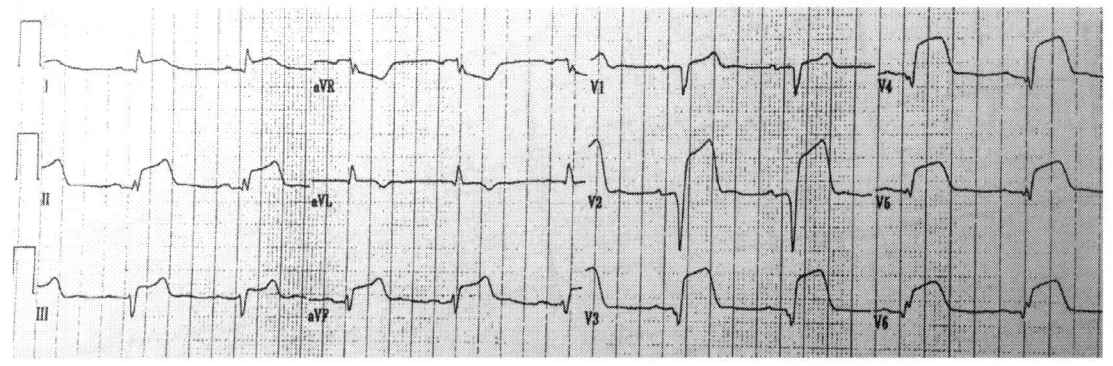

Fig. 70. Tombstone ST segments

important findings. This brings to mind the stages of evolution of the EKG in an untreated myocardial infarction:

A very early and transient sign of ischemia can be the isolated finding of peaked, very pointed T waves. By the way, this can also be seen with early hyperkalemia. ST elevation develops quickly and, in the first 24 hours, begins to subside. R waves start melting away (more about this later). Later, T waves begin to invert and Q waves develop. If an aneurysm forms, persistent and permanent ST elevation may occur.

As tissue necrosis occurs, it loses its ability to participate electrically. Its emitted signal is at first reduced so the leads overlying the infarct see less of a signal headed in their direction; the R waves get smaller. If the infarct is nontransmural, poor R wave amplitude in a group neighboring regional leads may be the permanent evidence. Any R wave left arises from the residual thinner living layer remaining of a once healthy full wall of myocardium. As has been previously discussed, it is important to point out that poor R wave progression in the early precordial and inferior leads may also be seen with left axis deviation i.e. in the absence of myocardial scar. If the main QRS axis is directed up and to the left, forces are drawn away from those leads; a beam headed to the far northeast leaves observers in the southwest somewhat in the dark.

If ischemic damage involves the full thickness of a wall, as in a completed transmural infarction, that zone sends no signal (dead men tell no tales). It behaves as a transparent window as far as the overlying leads are concerned so those leads, staring through the clear window, view the electrical signal on the wall of the heart that is directly opposite, heading outward and away from them. The genesis of Q waves as the permanent hallmark of transmural damage is thus explained.

A true posterior infarct which occurs from distal right coronary artery occlusion in most people has a special appearance. Recall about 10% of people have a larger-than-usual circumflex artery that supplies this zone. If that wall has infarcted, the anterior leads V1 and V2, positioned directly opposite the posterior wall, see normal anterior forces headed in their direction. However, there is no longer the usual posteriorly directed signal from the now-defunct posterior wall which ordinarily would oppose and "temper" the anterior wall's forward signal (but only a little because it is far away). The anterior signal is therefore exaggerated in amplitude from lack of competition. Taller than usual R waves in V1 and V2 may be seen as a result. Recall this was also seen in right ventricular hypertrophy. However, simply summarized, the explanations differ: tall R waves in V1 and V2 are due to loss of opposing forces in the case of a posterior scar. They are due to greater than usual anteriorly directed signal from more RV mass in the other.

The discussion turns to T waves and there are many similarities to ST segment depression regarding cause. While suggestive of ischemia, T inversion may also occur for other less critical reasons: LVH, LBBB, digoxin, hyperventilation and electrolyte disturbances such as hypokalemia.

As previously stated, T inversion is usual in lead aVR and sometimes seen as a normal phenomenon in other right sided leads such as V1 and lead III.

Rarely the inversion may extend to V2, termed "late transition of T wave polarity", a normal variant (in the absence of troubling signs and symptoms) which when present is likely to be so in younger adults.

When discussing ST depression, it was said that rapid upsloping or shallow depressions were generally less concerning than a deep and persistently depressed pattern unless the clinical picture was worrisome. ST elevation with an early repolarization swoosh pattern was less concerning than a tombstone pattern, also depending on coexisting signs and symptoms.

The same is true of T waves. The less worrisome form is an asymmetric wave, slow to descend and rapid to return to baseline, shown in Fig. 71. Often these findings accompany LVH (note the high voltage). It bears repeating that clinical correlation and comparison with old traces is essential when assessing such changes.

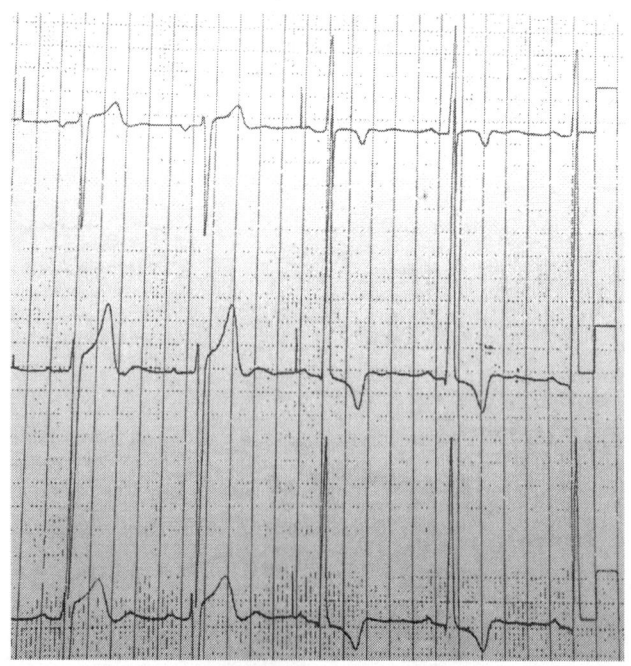

Fig. 71. Asymmetric T inversion

Biphasic T waves in multiple neighboring leads are more likely to represent true ischemia, especially if they develop acutely. They should also raise concern in a patient who cannot communicate but who is at risk for ischemia such as one who is intubated and critically ill with sepsis, shock or acidosis.

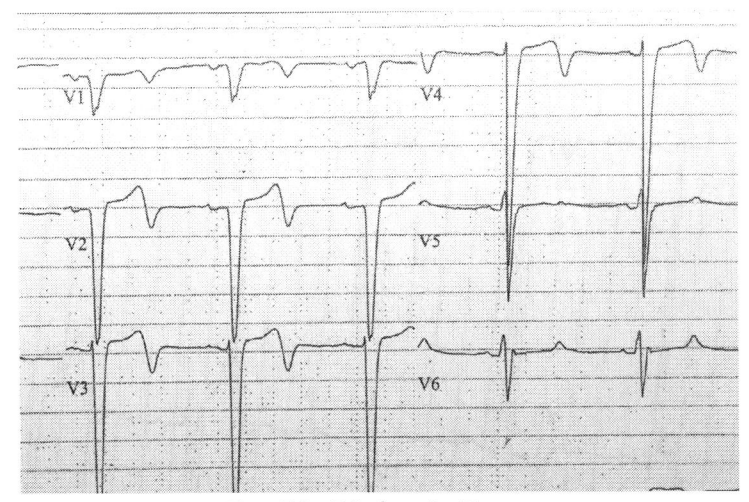

Fig. 72. Biphasic T waves

Symmetrically inverted T waves, especially those that are wide-mouthed, are also worrisome. These have the appearance of martini glasses. The wide mouth is due to prolonged QT interval. A variation can be deep symmetrical but narrow T waves that look like champagne flutes. In almost all cases these findings are accompanied by abnormal cardiac enzyme markers in the bloodstream.

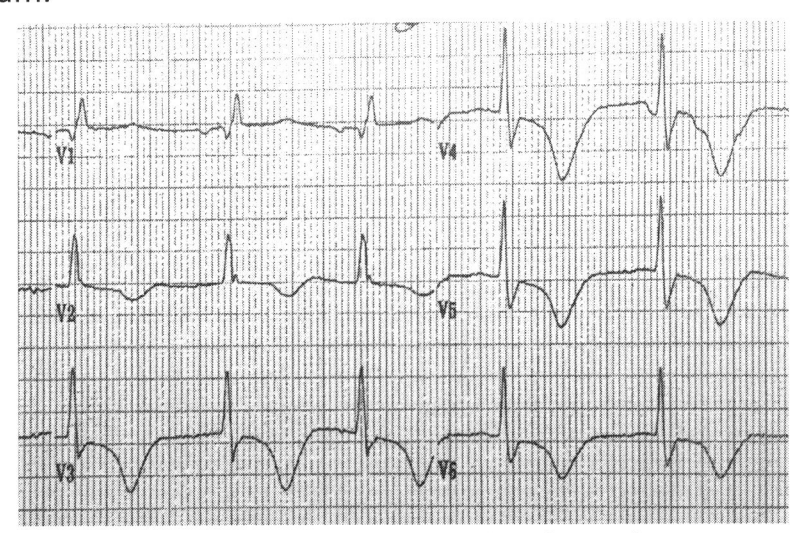

Fig. 73. Symmetric T inversion

In the early 1990's the cardiology department chairman of our hospital was retiring. He asked me to take over an EKG lecture he provided to medical school students rotating through our institution on a monthly basis. I asked his advice on topics and he told me he usually would teach each group how to use a marked plastic ruler distributed by a pharmaceutical company that helped measure the QT interval on an EKG. I mention this because from that invitation, I developed a more comprehensive set of talks presented to each group for the last few decades. These lectures are the basis for this book. It's ironic that we end discussing the QT interval, which was the seed for all of this, as the last topic, almost as an afterthought; but of course it is a critical topic.

Ideally, the heart should quickly and uniformly depolarize (contract) and repolarize (relax). If the heart relaxes in an uneven fashion, adjacent zones will find themselves at different levels of conductivity and refractory periods. This is a set-up for reentry as discussed at the start of Chapter 8. Many things can cause discrepant behavior between neighboring bits of tissue: regional ischemia, scar tissue, electrolyte disturbances, drug effects that affect some tissues more than others, microscopic zones of myocardial viral inflammation and even genetic defects of the ion channels controlling the action potential.

Without a clean move to an electrical baseline, small microscopic currents may continue to linger after relaxation was expected to have occurred. These are called afterpotentials, the equivalent of aftershocks following an earthquake. They prolong the QT duration because global electrical quiescence is delayed. The terminal QT represents a period of electrical instability when reentry is likely to happen. Like smoldering embers doused with gasoline, afterpotentials can explode if a strong electrical charge is applied, such as a premature ventricular contraction sparking at the end of the T wave when the microcurrents are most easily engaged. This is called an "R-on-T Phenomenon", R for the QRS wave of a PVC, T for the T wave of the preceding beat upon which the R falls. While uniform appearing ventricular tachycardia (VT) is possible, the classic arrhythmia of a prolonged QT is called "Torsades de Pointes" which translates to twisting around an axis.

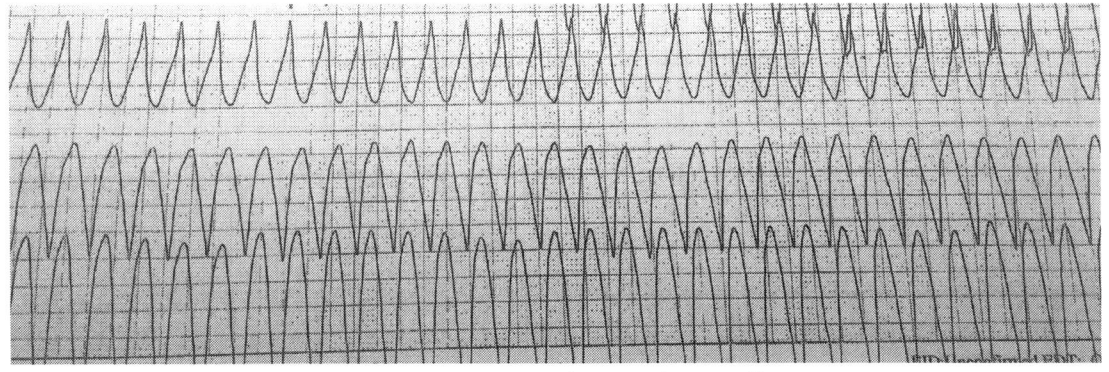

Fig. 74. Ventricular tachycardia

Uniform (or monomorphic) VT is seen in Fig 74. It has a consistent up and down appearance. It is like a stationary whirlpool rotating in the same spot and doesn't change appearance to an observer. Torsades is a very unstable rhythm that not only rotates but, like a tornado, moves about the landscape haphazardly so at times it appears to be approaching and at other times receding. As it changes direction, its angle of approach to a fixed EKG lead varies, so the QRS changes from up to neutral to down repeatedly, looking like spindles.

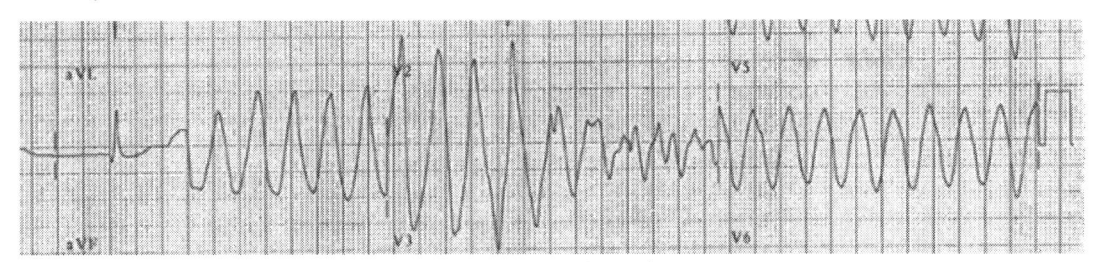

Fig. 75. Torsades-de-pointes

On the Torsades trace note how the rhythm starts with a downward spike landing on the first (and only) normal complex's T wave on the left side of the strip (R-on-T phenomenon).

Given the importance of the QT interval, how does one know if it is prolonged? The problem is that a QT measurement (start of QRS wave to end of T wave) is normally variable, related to heart rate. Its absolute measurement is shorter with increasing heart rate, longer with lowering heart rate. In order to standardize the interval, there is a concept called QTc which stands for corrected QT. Corrected to what? A heart rate of 60 bpm:

Take the heart rate on any tracing and measure its QT. Either by the calibrated plastic ruler I spoke of or by a program in the EKG machine's computer, a new corrected QT can be calculated which would match the original heart rate were it raised or lowered to 60 bpm. The high limit for a corrected QT is about 440 to 460 msec (higher end in women). For convenience, most EKG recordings do have that figure generated by the machine, along with rate, intervals and axis, displayed at the top of a trace.

What happens if a patient is on a simple cardiac monitor that doesn't generate these numbers and one must assess the QT? There is a simple rule. Whatever the heart rate, as long as it is reasonably regular (with atrial fibrillation there is too much beat to beat variation), the QT should be less than half the interval between any two successive beats. That means that if any heart rate is converted to 60 bpm (interval 1000 msec) the QT will correct to under half that (500 msec), close enough to the upper limit of normal of 460 msec.

And that's it. I sincerely hope you've finished this guide with a better understanding of EKG's. Every time an instructor points out an electrocardiographic finding and you realize "I know that already", I will be satisfied that I have achieved my goal. As time goes on there will be some subtle findings to be revealed that were beyond the scope of this book. But that is the nature of a career in medicine: the learning never stops.

Image credits:

Fig. 3 – Diagram of the Human Heart.svg.png, Author: Wapcaplet, Commons.Wikimedia.org, License: CC BY-SA 3.0

Fig. 4 – Conduction system of the heart without the heart-en.svg. Author: angelito7, Commons.Wikimedia.org, License: CC BY-SA 3.0

Fig. 5 – EKG Complex en.svg, Author: Hank van Helvete, derivative by hazmat2, March 4, 2014. Commons.Wikimedia.org, License: CC BY-SA 3.0

Fig. 9 – Limb leads of EKG.png, Author: Npatchett, March 27, 2015, Commons.Wikimedia.org, License: CC BY-SA 4.0

Fig. 10 – EKG leads.png, Author: Npatchett, March 27, 2015, Commons.Wikimedia.org, License: CC BY-SA 4.0

Fig. 12 – QRS Nomenclature.svg, Author: MoodyGroove, August 18, 2007, Commons.Wikimedia.org, License: CC BY-SA 3.0

Fig. 14 – QRS Axis, Author: Npatchett (modified by STeich), Commons.Wikimedia.org. License CC BY-3.0

Fig. 22 - Flight Around the World, Author: Jaen0000, Pixabay.com.

Fig. 24 – Right Ventricular Hypertrophy, Author: Michael Rosengarten, B Eng-MD, McGill, 2012, Commons.Wikimedia.org, License: CC BY-SA 3.0

Fig. 45 – Ventricular Fibrillation, amended from Jer5150, May 30, 2012, Commons-Wikimedia.org. License: CC BY-SA 3.0

Fig. 75 – Torsades-de-Pointes, amended by STeich from Jer5150, June 3, 2012, Commons-Wikimedia.org, License CC BY-SA 3.0

Index

A AIVR 54-56,58, Activation of ventricles 33-35 ,Adenosine 69, Afterpotentials 96, Alcohol 27, Anatomy, heart 8-9, conduction system 9-12, Amplitude 20, 27, Anti-arrhythmic drugs 40, Aorta 26, Atherosclerosis 82-86, Atrial fibrillation 60-62, Atrial Flutter 64, 68, 72, 74, AV Node Reentry Tachycardia 64, 68, 72,.

B Bachmann's Bundle 9, 10, Beta blockers 70, Bifascicular block 46, 80, Bigeminy 53, Bipolar leads 16, Biphasic P wave 30, Bundle branches 11, Bundle branch block 11,34, 42-44, 47, 56-57.

C Cardiomyopathy 27, Calcium channel blockers 70, Carotid message 70, Circulatory cycle 19, Clustering of leads 17, Couplet 52.

D Dance of 4 A's 86, Digoxin 56, 70, 79, 85, 93, diltiazem 70, 73.

E Early repolarization 88, Ectopic atrial rhythm 53, 54, Einstein 5, Einthoven 14, Einthoven's triangle 15, EKG paper 19. Electrical system supraventricular 47, ventricular 47-8.

F Fascicles 23, 33, First degree AV block 77.

G Gag reflex 70.

H Hemi block 23, 44-45, Hyperkalemia 41, 92, Hypertrophy 26, 27, 38-39, Hypokalemia 93.

I Ideoventricular rhythm12, 46, 55, 58, 81, Infra His block 77, Intervals, normal 29, Intraventricular conduction delay 39-40, Ischemia treatment 83.

J Junctional rhythm 11, 53, 57, 76, J point 85-86.

L Lyme's Disease 76

M Mobitz I 78, Mobitz II 80-81, Multifocal atrial tachycardia 59, myocarditis 27.

N Nomenclature of waves 21

P P biphasic 30,71, P mitrale 31, P pulmonale 29, PAC 49-53, PAT with block 79-80, Pericarditis 89-90, polarity defined 20, Posterior infarct 93, PR interval 11, Prolonged QT 96-97, Propafenone 73, Purkinje fibers 11, 47, PVC 51.

Q Q waves 92-93, QRS nomenclature 10, QT 95-96, QT corrected 98, Quinidine 40.

R R wave progression 37, R:S ratio 22-23, R-on-T 96, Rabbit ears 43,45, Reentry mechanism 63-64, Reperfusion rhythm 56, Rule of Deceleration 67, Rule of Rates 66.

S Saint Sebastian 13-14, Scar 37, Second degree AV block 78 Sinus arrhythmia 47-48, sinus tachycardia 67, ST depression 84, ST elevation 87, 90-91, Sotalol 40, Subendocardial ischemia 83-84,Supra His block 76.

T T waves 94-95, Tachy-brady syndrome 73, Tamponade 90, Teich's Law of Pulse Rate 73 , Third degree AV block 78-79, Torsades-de-Pointes 41, 97, Tombstone ST elevation 91-92 Transmural infarction 91, Transmural ischemia 86-87, Trifascicular block 46, 80, Trigeminy 53, Triplet 52.

U U wave 12, Unifascicular block 46, 80, Unipolar leads 16.

V V leads 16,17, Vagal tone 69-70, Valsalva maneuver 70, Vector 20, Ventricular fibrillation 62-65, Ventricular tachycardia 55, 66, 97, Verapamil 70, Vitruvian Man 13.

W Wandering atrial pacemaker 59, Wenckebach block 78, Wolf-Parkinson-White Syndrome 34, 44-45, 65, 66.

Stephen M Teich, M.D. received a B.A. in biology from the University of Rochester in 1974. He attended S.U.N.Y. Medical Center and trained in internal medicine at St. Vincent's Hospital and Medical Center in New York City. He became board certified in cardiology after a fellowship at the Washington D.C. Veterans' Hospital – Georgetown University program.

In 1983 he joined Abington Cardiology Associates at Abington Memorial Hospital in suburban Philadelphia, currently part of the Jefferson Health system, spending 33 years at that institution. While engaged in private practice, a great joy was teaching Abington residents, visiting house staff, students and cardiology fellows who rotated through from Temple, Jefferson and Drexel Schools of Medicine, Arcadia University's Physician Assistant Program and the Philadelphia College of Osteopathic Medicine.

During those decades, he developed a course in EKG interpretation and at the urging of his students translated his talks into this manuscript after leaving clinical medicine in 2016. He has received several awards for his teaching from students and residents, including the Golden Apple Award from Abington Memorial Hospital and the Blockley-Osler Award from Temple University School of Medicine. His peers in the Delaware Valley medical community have voted him an outstanding provider of cardiology care for the elderly population, as published in Philadelphia Magazine.

At the time of publication, he resides in suburban Philadelphia with his wife and two children. He continues to volunteer his teaching services at Abington Memorial Hospital and works at Caduceus Academy in Haverford, PA, tutoring medical students in physiology and pathology in preparation for national board examinations.

Made in the USA
Columbia, SC
29 July 2024